Jenny Ruhl

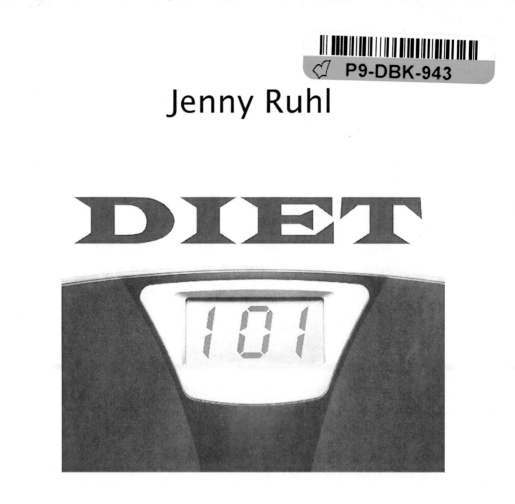

DIET

The Truth About Low Carb Diets

TECHNION Books

Published by Technion Books
P.O. Box 402
Turners Falls, MA 01376
technion@phlaunt.com

ISBN-13: 978-0-9647116-5-5
ISBN-10: 0-9647116-5-6

Table of Contents

Introduction

What made me think about writing this book was the invitation I received from Jimmy Moore in the spring of 2011 to do a podcast interview for his very popular "La Vida Low Carb" internet radio show. Though I'd considered writing about the low carb diet in the past, I'd held back, feeling that with so many other books available on the subject there was little I could add.

But the interview I did with Jimmy proved surprisingly popular with his large fandom and resulted in my being invited back to do second show. Many of the listeners who emailed me after hearing the podcasts told me that much of what I'd said about the science behind how low carb diets work was news to them and helped them deal with issues they'd run into with their diets. Even Jimmy said I'd told him things he hadn't known before.

At first I was surprised that this should be true, since he and his audience were such sophisticated, well-read, low carb dieters. But then I remembered that after I had spent a year on my first very low carb diet in 1998, I, too, had run into the same problems that derail the majority of those who attempt to follow these diets — even though I'd read all the bestselling books.

I wasn't completely new to low carb dieting when I'd started that diet. Like most people who reached their teens in the 1960s, I'd always known that the easiest way to lose weight was to cut out bread, potatoes, and desserts. Doing that periodically had kept my weight in the normal range. But a low carb diet had stopped being optional for me in 1998, when I received a diagnosis of diabetes after a year of relentless and ravenous hunger that had packed a sudden 30 lbs on my middle-aged, almost-menopausal body.

The book, *Dr. Bernstein's Diabetes Solution*, by Dr. Richard K. Bernstein taught me how important it was to maintain normal blood sugars. It explained that the best way to do this was to limit my daily carbohydrate intake to 36 grams. I ended up eating that way for 7 of the next 13 years. That kept my blood sugars normal, which made me enthusiastic about the diet. But after a heartening and dramatic loss of 20 lbs, which occurred over the first two months of my diet, I didn't lose another pound for the next two and a half years, even though I did all the things suggested in the bestselling low carb diet books.

It was only after I got a copy of Lyle McDonald's groundbreaking book, *The Ketogenic Diet*, that I learned for the first time what scientists knew about the changes very low carb diets make to our bodies. What I read in Lyle's book contradicted popular beliefs about the diet and helped me understand why my weight loss had stopped. He gave me the key concepts I needed to get my own diet working. I reached my goal weight in 2003 and have been maintaining at it ever since.

Lyle's book also showed me what treasures were hidden in the pages of dry, musty research journals. A few years later, when I realized that it was possible to read these scientific journals on the web, I started doing some research of my own.

I'd already earned a graduate degree in History, which had taught me how to read and evaluate published research and introduced me to the statistical techniques used in medical studies. I'd also spent years as a software developer, debugging complex, poorly documented systems—which turned out to be a good description of the human body. Over the years, friends who were more knowledgeable about biology explained the unfamiliar terms and concepts I encountered in academic medical research and pointed me to resources that gave me the background I needed to better understand them.

Eventually, my review of the published research about diabetes led me to numerous studies that made it very clear that the blood sugar levels that doctors believed to be normal were only normal if you considered heart attacks and nerve damage normal. In 2005 I put this information online on a web site, bloodsugar101.com. Over the years the site's traffic has doubled each year until by the end of 2011 it was receiving 1.5 million annual visitors.

Meanwhile I kept reading the latest medical research, including many small studies the health media paid no attention to. This is why I was able to warn my site's visitors that Avandia was causing heart problems and statins raising insulin resistance years before these stories hit the national press.

When I turned the information that was posted on my web site into a book and published it as *Blood Sugar 101: What They Don't Tell You About Diabetes* it became an Amazon bestseller, outranking many other books published by much larger mainstream publishers.

That's why, when the success of my podcasts made me think it might be time to write a book about low carb diets, I went back to the journals and carefully reread the studies that people in the low carb community usually cite as proving the safety and efficacy of the diet. As I had done when researching diabetes, I looked not only at what the studies concluded, but combed through the full text, hunting for the small nuggets of information buried in charts and tables that summaries don't mention.

I learned some fascinating things about glycogen, insulin, and hunger hormones that challenged my previous beliefs that glycogen accounted for only a very small amount of low carb weight loss and that the low carb diet worked better than other diets because it lowered insulin levels. I also discovered that even though, as I'd known, the low carb diet can greatly improve health, the way many people do the diet leaves them worse off than when they started. This gave me insight into why so many doctors still believe that low carb diets damage health.

Eventually the small bits of information buried in the texts of these research studies and reviews began to paint a fuller, more informative portrait of the real strengths and weaknesses of low carb diets. That more nuanced understanding is what I'll be sharing with you in the following chapters.

What you'll learn as we review the research is that people who have normal blood sugars can lose weight on any diet that limits their calories. But the reason so many people are willing to eat a diet that makes them give up so much of the foods they were raised with is that they *don't* have normal blood sugars. And because they don't, the low carb diet is the only diet that will keep them from being ravenously hungry.

Most people who find they can only lose weight on low carb diets, whether they know it or not, have blood sugars that fluctuate within a range that, while doctors call it normal, emphatically is not. Their blood sugars fall in the upper part of the normal range, but as I learned when I researched *Blood Sugar 101*, there's very strong evidence that people whose blood sugars fall into the higher end of the normal range run a much greater risk of developing heart disease. When I researched this book, I also learned that blood sugars surging up into that high normal range do things to our hunger hormones that make us more hungry.

The low carb diet generates so much enthusiasm in people whose blood sugars aren't entirely normal because it lowers blood sugar, which abolishes hunger and normalizes many factors associated with heart disease. But as you'll see, these improvements only last as long as you stick to the diet. And that's where the problems arise.

The research we'll examine makes it crystal clear that the classic low carb diets are too hard for most dieters to stick to over the long haul. And when they don't stick to their diets those former low carb dieters end up with worse health than they had before they started—even if they've managed to knock off a few pounds.

Fortunately, the same research shows that there's no need for most dieters to eat such stringent diets. Once you understand how your blood sugar works and, most importantly, once you understand how well your blood sugar is working, you can personalize your diet. You can cut out only the carbs your body can't handle. That will still silence your hunger and give you back your health.

When you've learned how to customize your diet, you can diet without having to exert heroic amounts of willpower each time you sit down at the dinner table. The diet that truly fits your own individual metabolic needs is the one diet you will be able to stick to—not for a month, or a year, but for life.

But before you can customize your diet, you'll need to put on your scientist hat and learn a bit more about how your body works, so you can understand what it was that stopped working that made you fat and what your uniquely tailored diet will have to do to fix it.

Blood sugar is the key to all of this, so you'll start out by learning what the phrase "blood sugar" really means. You'll learn how blood sugar works and what happens when it stops working. You'll learn why your own blood sugar may not be normal, even if the test the doctor ordered said it was.

You'll discover why slightly abnormal blood sugars cause the hunger that made you gain weight in the past and make it so hard to lose it now despite your good intentions. Because the best way to correct abnormal blood sugars is to cut down on your carbohydrate intake, next we'll take a close look at what happens to your body when you cut your carbs to different levels, from a modest decrease to the extremely low carb level that makes major changes in how your whole body works.

Once you understand this, we'll dig into the studies, and learn what they can teach us about how safe and effective low carb diets really are. We'll see how much weight people really lose on low carb diets, and how long it takes them to lose it. We'll learn how much carbohydrate they have to cut out to get the scale moving. We'll discover when and why most low carb dieters see their weight loss stall.

We'll also delve into the reasons why some low carb dieters lose weight but worsen their health, so that you can avoid the common mistakes they make that are common even among low carb dieters who succeed at losing weight and keeping it off.

Because the single most appealing feature of the low carb diet is the way it controls hunger, we'll take deeper look at how it affects the various hormones that stimulate and repress hunger. We'll see if scientific research can settle the controversies that rage over the diet, including whether it provides a "metabolic advantage" and lowers insulin resistance, or damages the kidneys and lowers thyroid hormones. We'll also investigate the claims of various supplements and functional foods to see if they really improve blood sugar and speed up weight loss.

There are some questions studies don't address, so occasionally I'll supplement what the studies can tell us with the results of some polls I've run over the past decade among people active in the online low carb diet and diabetes communities. Several of these polls were limited to people who had been successful in sticking to a low carb diet for three years or more. Their answers should prove very helpful if you'd like to follow in their footsteps.

If everything you've learned about the low carb diet comes from reading books written by people who are heavily invested in promoting it, some of what you will read here will surprise you. Some common claims made about the low carb diet do not hold up to scrutiny, including the idea that it works by lowering insulin levels and eliminating insulin resistance.

If you've been sold the idea that the low carb diet is the ideal human diet for everyone, you may be surprised to learn that this is far from true and that plenty of people lose weight and greatly improve their health on moderate and even high carbohydrate diets.

Perhaps the most unusual claim you will find documented in this book is this: The only people for whom the low carb diet is truly necessary are those who have abnormal blood sugars, whose numbers are ballooning, not because of poor lifestyle choices, as you've been told, but because of a hidden epidemic of poisoning caused by toxic industrial and agricultural chemicals that permeate our air, water, and food supply.

The impact of these toxins, which is already bad enough, has been worsened by the detrimental effects of several commonly prescribed pharmaceutical drugs that research clearly shows cause both abnormal blood sugars and obesity. Because abnormal blood sugars cause hunger, the victims of this damage *do* overeat, and that overeating can make them very fat, but that overeating is the result, not the cause, of the damage that this perfect storm of toxic exposures has done to their bodies.

We'll take a good look at research that documents all this, and some of it may come as a shock to you. The poisons that are driving the obesity epidemic are rarely mentioned in the media because the companies that sell those toxic products and the media who advertise them would prefer that you blame yourself for making poor food choices rather that learn that your body has sustained permanent damage from exposure to products you were told were safe and healthy.

Once you've reviewed this research, it will be time to put your new knowledge to work. You'll learn how to use a powerful tool you can buy at the drugstore to find out how damaged your own blood sugar might be. With that knowledge, you'll be able to make your own informed decisions as to what kind of diet is best for you.

If you choose a low carb diet, using the technique you'll learn here, you'll no longer have to rely on the word of distant experts to know how low to drop your carbohydrate intake to control your appetite, lose weight, and improve your health.

You'll also read insights contributed by dieters who have managed to stay on their low carb diets for three years or more. Their advice will not only show you what it takes to lose weight on a low carb diet, but what it takes to maintain the weight you lose.

We'll go through the list of the troubling side effects that are reported by many low carb dieters and learn the not-always obvious ways of addressing them. You'll find out why you don't have to smell bad to lose weight, and why, in fact, the dragon breath so often associated with very low carb diets can be a sign that you're doing the diet wrong.

Then we'll take a hard look at stalls. We'll discuss the tried and true strategies that help people break through them. But we'll also draw on insights from cutting edge research that suggest that sometimes a stall is your body's way of telling you that any further dieting will make it impossible to maintain the weight you've already lost.

Throughout the text you'll find citations to research studies. These are given in parentheses with the name of the first author of the study followed by its publication date. You'll find an alphabetical list of the cited articles along with their URLs in the References section at the end of the book.

I provide these citations because I don't expect you to believe something I say just because I tell you to. I grew up as part of the generation whose motto was "question authority," so I don't lay down the law. I just give you the information and tools you need to evaluate the claims you read, trusting you to make your own decisions.

Nowhere in this book will I tell you what kind of low carb diet is best or lecture you on what to eat. I believe very strongly that the best diet is the one you can stick to. My years interacting with thousands of dieters online have taught me that each person's physiology varies in subtle but important ways from that of everyone else. So the diet that is right for you may not be the diet that is right for me, or Jimmy Moore, or anyone whose genes, personality, and metabolism differ from ours.

All blood sugar measurements used in this book are given in the kind of units used in the United States: mg/dl. All weights are reported in pounds. Since most researchers report blood sugars in mmol/L, and report weight in kilograms, when discussing studies I've translated the units they use into the units used in the United States when necessary. Readers from parts of the world that use the other units can convert mg/dl values to mmol/L by dividing the mg/dl value by 18. To convert pounds to kilograms, divide them by 2.2.

I've had a lot of fun researching and writing this book. I hope you take as much pleasure in reading it. But that's enough introduction. Now it's time to dive in and learn what the term "blood sugar" really means and why the way that our blood sugars fluctuate when we eat carbs creates the subtle but relentless hunger that drives so many of us to eat the foods that makes us fat.

Chapter 1
Hunger and Your Not So Normal Blood Sugar

If it weren't for hunger, losing weight would be easy.

If you could just eat less food than your body needs, it would have no choice but to burn the excess fat you've stored. For that matter, if it weren't for hunger, you wouldn't need to lose weight. If your interest in food shut down when you'd eaten enough to supply your energy needs for the day, the feedback loops and hormone messaging systems that regulate our metabolisms would have kept your weight stable, without you having to give it a second thought.

Many people's bodies work just that way. We call them "normal people." A typical normal person will maintain a weight within a pound or two over the course of an entire year without paying any attention to how much they're eating. If they eat too much, the exquisitely tuned systems that maintain metabolic balance will raise the rate at which they burn calories or lower their interest in eating. If they eat too little, their metabolisms will slow and hunger will kick in until they've eaten enough to replace the body fat they've burned.

But if you're reading this book, the chances are good this isn't the way *your* body works. Because you keep wanting to eat even when you have enough fat stored to get you through months—or years—of starvation. And when you try to cut back on your intake, that urge becomes even stronger, eventually overcoming your best intentions.

If you are already eating a low carb diet, the relentless hunger you experienced when you ate other diets may have convinced you that the low carb diet is the only diet for you. Many people who have been tormented by an uncontrollable urge to eat find that the low carb diet curbs their hunger. After only a few days of cutting down on their carbohydrate intake, they suddenly, and sometimes for the first time in their adult lives, reclaim control over their eating. They discover it wasn't a personal weakness, greed, or gluttony that drove them to eat in the past, but something else—something that happens only when they eat carbohydrates. Now the hunger that kept them from being able to diet disappears—as long as they keep their carbs low.

At this point, many people decide they are "carbohydrate addicts," demonize carbohydrates, and proclaim that they will never again let evil carbs cross their lips. The belief that carbs are evil may be reinforced the first time they go off their diet, too, when six or seven pounds come back in a single day, along with a raging hunger so intense it makes it almost impossible to get back onto the diet.

After that happens, the dieter who goes back on a low carb diet may do so with an added burden of fear. Their diet is no longer a choice, it's a life sentence, and severe punishment awaits them if they transgress. Though they may stay on their diet, for many the joy has gone out of it. Meanwhile, the weight loss that motivated them to start the diet comes to a stop, often leaving them far heavier than they had hoped to be, while the restrictions the diet requires continue, keeping them from joining friends and family in the many food-related events that make up their social life. Eventually, a majority of those who embarked with such hope on a low carb diet decide they are doomed to be fat and quit.

It doesn't have to be that way. But to keep this from happening, you need to understand what exactly the low carb diet does: how it silences the hunger signal and why the way it does that makes the pounds drop off at first and come right back any time you go off the diet.

The Low Carb Diet Lowers Blood Sugar

What exactly does the low carb diet do that other diets don't? Why is it so effective for eliminating hunger, and why does hunger rebound so strongly when you go off it? The answer to both questions is that the low carb diet lowers how high your blood sugar rises after you eat.

Hunger is triggered by falling blood sugars, for reasons we'll explain shortly. But for sugars to fall they must first rise, and what pushes them up is the sugar and starch you eat. The low carb diet's most powerful effect derives from the way that it stops blood sugars from rising, which keeps them from dropping in the way that triggers hunger. No steeply falling blood sugar, no hunger. It's as simple as that.

Though you may have heard that it is high insulin levels that cause you to become hungry when you eat carbs, even people who make *lower* than normal levels of circulating insulin, like myself, experience hunger if we eat enough carbs to send out blood sugar shooting up and rushing down.

And the faster our blood sugars fall and the steeper the drop, the hungrier we get. Just how hungry plummeting blood sugars can make you is indicated by the story that was posted by a woman with Type 1 diabetes on an online discussion board. She'd woken up in the middle of the night in the midst of an episode of very low blood sugar so hungry that she tried to eat her alarm clock.

Most of us will never become that hungry, because our blood sugars won't ever drop that fast or that low. But while we won't experience the kind of dramatic episode that makes for a good story, we *will* get hungry every time our blood sugar drops, with hunger coming on, often quite subtly, an hour or two after we eat. This keeps us snacking throughout the day, even though starchy and sugary snacks send our blood sugar up and down again, which makes us even hungrier.

But the Doctor Says My Blood Sugar Is Normal!

Many of you reading this may be thinking, "This can't apply to me. My doctor told me my blood sugar was normal." And I don't doubt that for a minute, because doctors also assured me that my blood sugar was normal even when, after taking a single course of a medication that turns out to damage blood sugar metabolism, I suddenly developed a raging hunger of a kind I'd never before experienced in my 48 years of life. A year later, a smart doctor tested my blood sugar after breakfast — in her office with a meter — and discovered I was fully diabetic, but the standard screening tests I'd been given throughout the previous year had all shown normal values.

That was what set me on my quest to research the question of what is a truly normal blood sugar. And what I learned when I reviewed hundreds of pieces of laboratory research was that the criteria that doctors use to evaluate their patients' blood sugars treat blood sugars as normal while they are high enough to wreak havoc on our organs.

That this is true is shown by the research finding that on the day when they are diagnosed, almost half the people who receive a diabetes diagnosis already have medical conditions that are caused only by years of exposure to high blood sugars. (Spijkerman, 2003)

Take for example, heart disease. Though you are often told that your cholesterol level is the best predictor of future heart disease, this is not true. As we'll see in Chapter 6, several large epidemiological studies have demonstrated that the result of a simple blood sugar test called the A1C test tracks much more closely to the risk of developing heart disease than any cholesterol test. These studies also document that the incidence of heart disease starts to rise in people whose A1C test results cross a threshold that is well within the range doctors have been taught is completely normal. (BS101: A1C)

Another blood sugar-related symptom that occurs in this supposedly "normal range" is the onset of tendon problems like carpal tunnel syndrome and frozen shoulder. Research shows that people who develop these problems are more likely than others to be diagnosed with diabetes ten years after they develop their tendon problem. This is because these problems are caused by blood sugars that, though doctors consider them normal, are high enough to damage the fragile capillaries that supply our tendons. (BS101: Tendons)

It is when blood sugars rise into the upper part of the normal range where this damage starts to happen that hunger problems also begin. But to really understand why this happens, we need to know a bit more about what we mean when we talk about blood sugar.

What *Is* Blood Sugar?

You have sugar floating around in your bloodstream, right now. Real live sugar, exactly like the sugar that you find in candies like Sweetarts. That sugar is called dextrose in the U.S. and glucose everywhere else. This glucose is what nutritionists call a simple sugar, to distinguish it from other sugars that are made up by linking simple sugars like glucose and fructose together to form a larger molecule.

Glucose, like all simple sugars, it is made up of a backbone of carbon to which are attached hydrogen and oxygen molecules, in a pattern that ensures there are always two hydrogen molecules for each oxygen molecule present. This is the same ratio that we find in water, which is why sugar is called a *carbohydrate*. (The term *hydrate* is used in chemistry to describe a solid substance that contains hydrogen and oxygen in the same proportion as water.)

Your tissues are full of other kinds of sugars, and these sugars are essential to building vital structures like your cell membranes. Some of these complex sugars must be present in your cells for those cells to synthesize essential proteins correctly. But none of these other sugars plays the role that glucose does, because the glucose that floats around in your bloodstream is essential to keeping you alive.

It is this glucose in our bloodstreams that we refer to as *blood sugar*, and the reason it must circulate in our blood at all times is because it is the essential fuel some cells deep within our brains depend on for the energy that lets them go about their various functions.

Getting Your Brain Its Glucose is Job One

This is the central truth that drives metabolism. Except for the hard-working neurons in your brain, most other cells in your body can and do burn another kind of fuel when glucose gets scarce—fat. It's to provide this alternative fuel that fat also circulates in your bloodstream, in the form of triglycerides, which you may recognize as being one of the lipids that is measured when you have your cholesterol tested. But those critical cells in your brain that keep you conscious can not burn fat, because fatty acids can't cross the blood-brain barrier.

Though your brain only weights about 3 lbs and represents 2% or less of your total body weight, it burns 25% of all the glucose your body burns. Much of that is used to keep you conscious. Your brain cells are so dependent on their supply of glucose that, if there is ever less than 30 milligrams of glucose in each deciliter of your blood, your brain will start to shut down in a desperate attempt to keep you alive.

When this starts to happen, your visual field may blank out on one side, or you may start seeing flashing lights. You'll become confused and possibly hostile and combative. Eventually your vision may shut down completely. If your liver doesn't respond to the brain's distress signals by dumping stored glucose into your bloodstream you're likely to go into a coma since a comatose brain needs only 55% as much glucose as one that is conscious. (Laureys, 2004)

The longer you remain in a coma induced by glucose deprivation, the more likely you are to experience permanent brain damage. If the coma goes on long enough, eventually you die. (The Merck Manuel: Hypoglycemia)

This sounds frightening, so you might wonder why it isn't on the long list of health issues you've been told to worry about. The answer is that unless some catastrophic event stops your blood from circulating to your brain or you inject an abnormally high dose of insulin it never happens.

This glucose supply to the brain is so essential that your body has evolved backup systems and backup systems to those backup systems to ensure that there is always enough glucose circulating in your body to keep your brain functioning.[1]

How Much Glucose Do You Need?

All of the starches you eat, and most of the complex sugars, can be

---

[1] The coma we just described is often called a "diabetic coma" and is most likely to occur after a person accidentally injects a massive dose of insulin which removes all the glucose from their bloodstream. It is a common and deadly misunderstanding to think that a person in such a coma needs insulin. Injecting insulin into a person in this kind of diabetic coma can kill them.

The appropriate response is to inject glucagon, a hormone that invokes one of the body's fail-safe systems and caused glucose to quickly enter the bloodstream. Since a coma also results when some people with diabetes develop extremely high blood sugars that do require insulin injections, the appropriate response if you find a person with diabetes in a coma is to call an ambulance and let professionals determine the right injection.

broken down via digestion to provide glucose. And because all the other cells in your body can also burn fat if glucose supplies drop, it doesn't take much glucose to keep your brain happy. You only need to maintain a minimum of 70 milligrams of glucose in every deciliter of blood at all times for everything to run smoothly. (This glucose concentration is abbreviated as 70 mg/dl.)

Since most people have between 5 and 6 liters of blood in their body, or 50 to 60 deciliters, a person who weighs 150 lbs will have roughly 4 grams of glucose in their bloodstream when their blood sugar level is 70 mg/dl. That's as much glucose as you'd find in a single small piece of hard candy.

People who are heavier will have more sugar in their blood, with the exact amount depending on their size. Since they have more blood circulating, it takes more glucose to keep the concentration up. But a person who weighs 300 lbs won't need to have more than 8 grams of glucose in their blood at any given time.

Of course, a person needs to ingest more than just that 4 to 8 grams of glucose each day because at every moment some of this glucose is being taken up by their cells and burned. How much? It varies, because our bodies switch back and forth between burning glucose and fat throughout the day.

Studies of people who were fasting suggest that under normal conditions the amount of glucose needed to supply your neurons is between 110 and 145 grams a day. (Owen, 1967) That works out to 4 to 6 grams an hour. You could get that 100 grams of glucose by eating only the carbohydrate contained in four slices of commercially baked white bread, since the starch they contain is easily digested back into glucose.

And if you can't find four slices of toast one day? Don't worry. Your brain will fall back on a reserve of carbohydrate your liver keeps handy. It stores glucose in the form of a starchy substance called *glycogen*. Your body tops up this supply any time you eat more carbohydrate than you need to supply that day's quota of blood sugar.

Glycogen Is Your Emergency Glucose Supply

Glycogen is interesting stuff, and you have to understand how it works to fully comprehend how the low carb diet affects your weight. Though glycogen is starchy, it's different from the starch stored by plants like potatoes or wheat. Plant starch is nothing more than a long chain of glucose molecules bonded together. But animals have evolved a more complex molecule to warehouse the glucose they can't use immediately.

This animal glycogen is made up of a protein core to which are attached many long, branching chains of glucose. Each glycogen molecule can contain up to 30,000 glucose molecules chained together, all of which can be swiftly converted back into individual glucose molecules with the help of three separate enzymes. (Wikipedia: Glycogen)

Glycogen is what your body uses to store glucose that can be accessed immediately when there's a critical need for it, like when your blood sugar is dropping. Think of it as the "quick release" form of glucose storage.

There are two main places where your body stores glycogen: your liver and your muscles.[2] The glycogen stored in your muscles is only for the use of the muscle cells themselves. It's burned when you need to generate a potentially life-saving burst of speed. The glycogen used to supply the glucose used by your neurons is stored in your liver.

Conventional estimates, based largely on research conducted on extracted rat livers in the 1950s and '60s, suggest that the liver of the average person should hold between 100 and 150 grams of glycogen — 5 ounces — which is, not so coincidentally, enough to keep your brain running for an entire day. (e.g. Van der Vies, 1953)

If your diet isn't supplying enough extra glucose to let your liver store glycogen, your body has several more tricks up its sleeve that will provide your brain with that vital glucose. If they have to, the liver and kidneys can synthesize glucose out of protein and, to a much lesser extent, fat via a process called *gluconeogenesis*, which we'll discuss further in Chapter 2.

But for now the important thing to understand that as far as your body is concerned, keeping enough glucose circulating in your bloodstream to keep the brain going is Job One. And because it is so essential, any threat to the integrity of the brain's glucose supply, no matter how slight, sets off alarms that trigger immediate action. You're very familiar with one way the brain triggers that action: it generates your old enemy, the hunger signal.

The most common threat that produces a hunger signal is a swift, downward trend in the amount of glucose in your blood. This makes sense. If your blood sugar is plummeting, there's no way of knowing when, or even *if*, it will stop. So the safest response to a swift drop in blood sugar is to replace any other, more trivial thoughts with the single command, "Eat! Carbs! Now!"

---

[2] Recent research has revealed that your brain also stores a very small amount of glycogen in cells called astrocytes, which it draws on in hypoglycemic emergencies. But this supply only provides 20 minutes worth of glucose. (Brown, 2007)

This doesn't happen very often when a person's blood sugar works the way it's designed to, which is why normal people have such a tough time understanding how hard it is for people whose blood sugar is *not* normal to control their food intake. But very early in the process by which people's blood sugar control starts to deteriorate, the way that blood sugar behaves *will* trigger that hunger signal every time a person eats a meal that contains more carbohydrate than they can handle.

To understand this better, let's take a closer look at how a normal person's blood sugar levels vary throughout the day and how that pattern changes when people's blood sugar stops being entirely normal.

How Normal People's Blood Sugar Fluctuates

In a normal person, blood sugar levels oscillate within a narrow range throughout the day. They rise after meals, as glucose from digested carbohydrates enters the bloodstream. Then they quickly drop back to normal within an hour or two, as cells take up that glucose to burn for fuel or store as glycogen for future use.

The liver converts any excess glucose that remains in the bloodstream after a meal into glycogen, unless its glycogen stores have been topped up. Then the liver transforms the rest of its excess glucose into the other kind of molecule it uses to store the energy bound up in glucose: fat.

Fat molecules are far more compact than glycogen, and take up much less room, which makes fat ideal for long-term energy storage. But fat has one disadvantage compared to glycogen. The reason it's more compact is that the liver makes fat by removing 9/10ths of the oxygen that was in the original glucose molecule, leaving little behind but hydrogen and carbon. As a result, 9/10ths of the fat you store can't be converted back to glucose. So stored fat can't be utilized by your brain in a crisis when blood sugars fall.

Obviously, it would be best, from the standpoint of your metabolism, to avoid storing precious glucose as fat if at all possible. That's why it lets your blood sugar rise after meals, to distribute as much of the glucose that came in with your meals to your muscles so they can store it away as glycogen.

But because blood sugar levels only slightly higher than normal are toxic to your organs, healthy people's bodies don't let their blood sugar rise more than a small amount after meals. As soon as they hit the threshold over which damage might occur, their pancreases secrete enough insulin to bring their blood sugar back down into the safe zone.

The Pattern of Truly Normal Blood Sugar

Figure 1 shows how, on average, the concentration of blood sugar rises and falls throughout the day in a normal person. In this example the person has eaten a high carbohydrate meal containing roughly 90 grams of carbohydrate at 8 AM, Noon, and 6 PM, followed by a snack containing 30 grams of carbohydrate eaten at 8 PM.

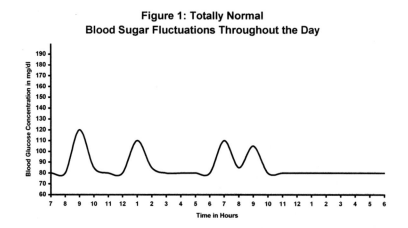

**Figure 1: Totally Normal
Blood Sugar Fluctuations Throughout the Day**

The blood sugar values you see on this graph are based on those reported in a study of normal people whose blood sugars were monitored over many hours by a device called a Continuous Glucose Monitoring System. It used an implanted needle to sample their blood every few minutes after they ate a high carbohydrate breakfast. The values you see here represent the *average* reading in this group of normal people.

I have extrapolated the readings for the rest of the daily meals from their breakfast readings. They are slightly lower than the readings at breakfast time because everyone, including, normal people, becomes slightly more insulin resistant when they have just woken up. This is why most people experience their highest blood sugar readings of the day after breakfast. (Christiansen, 2006)

As you can see, even after eating a starchy, sugary breakfast, this normal person's blood sugar doesn't rise over 120 mg/dl. That appears to be the threshold that truly normal people never exceed for more than a very brief time. People with diabetes who have used their blood sugar meters to test their normal friends and family have verified that many of them never test over 120 mg/dl at any time after a meal.

The reason that blood sugar levels higher than this are reported in every study of supposedly normal people is that the people selected for these studies are considered normal because their *fasting blood glucose* or A1C test result falls within the normal range. But it turns out that neither of these tests tells us how their blood sugars behave after a meal. Many people still have completely normal *fasting* glucose and A1C test results long after their post-meal blood sugars have risen to heights that enhance their likelihood of developing early diabetic complications. (BS101: Misdiagnosis)[3]

The belief that *truly normal* blood sugars rarely rise over 120 mg/dl is reinforced by the finding that many "diabetic" complications start to become more frequent when people's blood sugar spends any significant amount of time over 140 mg/dl. (BS101: Research)

The scale of this chart goes up to 200 mg/dl. If you take a glucose tolerance test, that is how high your blood sugar would have to remain for *two whole hours* before most doctors would tell you that you were diabetic.[4]

The Pattern Doctors Consider Mildly Abnormal

Figure 2 on Page 22 shows the pattern of blood sugars most doctors would consider only "mildly abnormal." A person whose blood sugar behaved like this would be told they had *prediabetes*. But because doctors rarely order the expensive glucose tolerance test that would uncover this pattern, most people who have prediabetes are unaware that they have it.

You won't be diagnosed as "prediabetic" by most doctors until your blood sugar stays over 140 mg/dl for two whole hours after the start of a glucose tolerance test or until your fasting glucose is higher than 100 mg/dl. Many people's fasting blood glucose won't rise that high until their post-meal readings have been reaching prediabetic levels day in and day out, for years. Some older doctors won't consider you

---

[3] How bad a job the A1C does at diagnosing prediabetes and diabetes becomes clear when you learn of the findings of a study of 4,706 people who had received both A1C tests and glucose tolerance tests. When the researchers gave A1C tests to people who had been diagnosed using a glucose tolerance test, they found the A1C test "... missed 70% of individuals with diabetes, 71–84% with dysglycemia [milder abnormal blood sugars], and 82–94% with pre-diabetes." (Olsen, 2010)

[4] According to the American Diabetes Associations document, "Diagnosis and Classification of Diabetes Mellitus," a random reading over 200 mg/dl is also diagnostic of diabetes, but most doctors ignore this. (ADA: Criteria)

to be prediabetic until your fasting blood sugar reaches over 110 mg/dl or even 125 mg/dl, as the diagnostic cutoff for prediabetes has been revised downward several times since 1998.

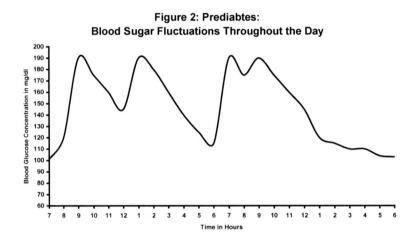

Figure 2: Prediabtes:
Blood Sugar Fluctuations Throughout the Day

Notice how much more steeply this person's blood sugar rises and falls compared to the blood sugar of a normal person. The long downward slides you see on the graph tend to be accompanied by hunger, as the brain has no way of knowing if that steep slope will continue downward until there is no more glucose left to keep it functioning, so it triggers the hunger alarm to ensure the person eats enough carbohydrate to prevent that from happening.

However, the worse blood sugar gets, the longer it takes to decline from its peak. So the person with this abnormal pattern of prediabetic blood sugars may actually not be as hungry after meals as they used to be, back when their blood sugar was still considered normal.

Back then they were likely to be experiencing a third pattern of blood sugar fluctuation throughout the day that is even more likely to get the brain sending out hunger signals, meal after meal. You'll see that pattern in Figure 3.

The High Normal Blood Sugar Pattern that Causes Hunger

The blood sugar pattern you'll see in Figure 3 on Page 23 is considered 100% normal by doctors. These values, in fact, come from the same study we used to construct the graph in Figure 1 that showed you a completely normal blood sugar pattern. But the values graphed in Figure 3 are those recorded by the individuals in this group of normal people whose blood sugars were nearing the top of the normal range, though they still remained completely within it.

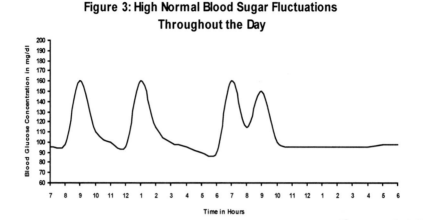

Figure 3: High Normal Blood Sugar Fluctuations Throughout the Day

Two hours after eating, their blood sugar was well under the 140 mg/dl level doctors consider to be the beginning of the abnormal range. Nor, as you can see, did they drop at any time into the range doctors would diagnose as abnormally low or *hypoglycemic*, which is the range under 70 mg/dl (though some of the other supposedly normal people in this study did, in fact, register values in that range.)[5]

Doctors know that blood sugars that drop into the hypoglycemic range can trigger a dramatic hunger response along with a sudden release of adrenaline that gets your heart racing, your pulse pounding, and, most importantly, your liver converting glycogen into glucose.

---

[5] Hypoglycemia is another blood sugar pattern that is often found in insulin resistant people who have the genes that predispose them to become fully diabetic as they age. It happens when their pancreases secrete a burst of insulin to bring their blood sugars down after eating. Because they are insulin resistant their cells don't respond quickly to the insulin so their blood sugar continues to climb. This leads to the secretion of even more insulin. Eventually all the insulin secreted kicks in and this ends up lowering their blood sugar so much that it drops below 70 mg/dl, into the range that the brain, rightly, considers an emergency.

Over time, as these people's ability to secrete insulin declines, their blood sugars start rising higher after meals and no longer plunge to the hypoglycemic level. Because their blood sugars no longer sink to the level of true hypoglycemia, they stop getting the bursts of stress hormone that occur when people are truly hypoglycemic, so they feel better. Many interpret this as a sign that their health has improved. In fact, it is getting worse, and they are still likely to be experiencing the steep declines after eating that increase hunger.

Your liver dumps this glucose into your bloodstream almost immediately to push your blood sugar back up into the safe range.

What they don't know, because it is a much more subtle effect observed mostly by those of us who use blood sugar meters to closely monitor our diabetic blood sugars, is that a fast, steep drop of this kind, which occurs when blood sugars remain above the hypoglycemic range, will *also* affect the brain's "watch that glucose level!" warning centers, though this reaction isn't as extreme as the true hypoglycemic attack.

What this means is that when your blood sugars drop 60 mg/dl in a single hour, rather than the 35 mg/dl that is truly normal, you aren't likely to start sweating or to feel as if you're going to pass out the way you would if you were experiencing a true hypoglycemic attack. But your brain will send out a burst of the hormones that tell you to go find some carbs to eat, just to be sure that your blood sugar doesn't keep dropping at that same, steep, scary rate. If it did, your blood sugar would quickly drop into the zone that threatens the brain's precious glucose supply.

That the downward slide actually bottoms out at a safe level means nothing to the brain, because it is while that steep slide is *occurring* that it sends out the hunger signal. There is too much at stake to take a "wait and see" approach.

People whose blood sugars go up and down this way, even though they fluctuate in the normal range, have to exert enormous amounts of self-control to get through a day without overeating, because after each meal their brains send out hunger signals that take over their consciousness and make them feel a strong need to keep feeding.

It is also why truly normal people are so judgmental of people who have trouble controlling their weight. Because a normal person does *not* have that brain-mediated hunger signal clanging away and doesn't think about food obsessively, the way someone does whose blood sugar is riding this kind of rollercoaster.

If you get extremely hungry when you eat meals containing normal amounts of carbohydrate, you don't have to take my word about it that your blood sugar is likely to be spiking this way. You can test it yourself, at home. We'll show you how in Chapter 9.

Points to Remember from This Chapter:

1. The low carb diet is effective because it limits the blood sugar fluctuations that cause hunger.

2. Truly normal blood sugars stay under 120 mg/dl at all times.

3. Many people who are told they have normal blood sugars don't. Their blood sugars go high enough to dramatically increase their hunger and cause health problems.

4. Much of the work of our metabolism involves ensuring that the brain always gets the steady supply of glucose that keeps you conscious.

4. Hunger is a response to steep drops in blood sugar, even those within the normal range, that trigger the brain's protective systems that ensure it gets a constant supply of glucose.

Chapter 2
What Happens When You Cut Carbs

Now that you know something about the different ways blood sugar can behave after you eat carbs, it's time to take an in-depth look at what happens when you cut down on carbohydrates.

Cutting Carbs When Blood Sugar Is Normal

If your blood sugar is truly normal, when you cut down on your carbohydrate intake very little happens.

Let's say your usual lunch is a hamburger on a bun served with four ounces of french fries and a glass of milk. This meal contains about 100 grams of carbohydrates, one third of the amount most nutritionists would recommend you eat every day. Since you are normal, after you eat it, your blood sugar rises no higher than 120 mg/dl and then quickly drops back under 100 mg/dl.

If you were to eat the hamburger without its bun, you'd be eating 25 grams less carb. So you'd have eliminated one quarter of all the carbohydrate in your meal. Cut out the glass of milk, and you've removed another 20 grams of carb. Your meal now contains 45% less carbohydrate than usual. But if you or any truly normal person wore a continuous glucose monitor, the blood sugar curve you'd see after deducting those 45 grams from your meal wouldn't be much different from the one we showed you in Figure 1 where the subjects were eating a high carbohydrate meal containing 100 grams of carbohydrate.

That's because, the body of a normal person handles 25 grams of carbohydrate the same way it handles 100 grams. In both cases, as soon as you lay eyes on your meal you start to secrete insulin. Then, once you digest between 8 and 16 grams of glucose—the exact amount depends on your body size—your blood sugar starts to rise until it approaches 120 mg/dl.

That's not very far from the range over 140 mg/dl where glucose begins to become toxic. But since you are normal, as soon as your blood sugar nears this level, sensors in your pancreas detect it and stimulate your pancreas to secrete another big dollop of insulin. By the time the rest of the glucose from your meal reaches your bloodstream, there is enough insulin circulating in your blood to push every glucose molecule into cells that will burn it, store it as glycogen, or stash what you can't burn right away in the form of fat.

That's why a normal person's blood sugar would rise to around 120 whether they ate 100 grams of carb, 50 grams, or 25 grams. Then it would drop right down. If you are truly normal, the only way you can change the way your blood sugar behaves after meals is to cut your carbohydrate intake down to an extremely low level, so low your blood sugar doesn't even approach 120 mg/dl. For most people that will happen when they eat a meal containing between 8 and 15 grams of carbs. When they do that their blood sugar will rise only a little bit after they eat.

You can see the impact of cutting carbs on a normal person illustrated in Figure 4. The thick line shows how their blood sugar would rise and fall were they to eat only 8-15 grams of carbohydrate. The thin line shows what would happen if they ate enough carbohydrate to push their blood sugar up to around 120 mg/dl.

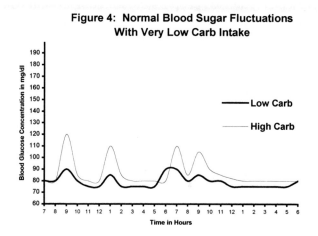

Figure 4: Normal Blood Sugar Fluctuations With Very Low Carb Intake

But even if a normal person cut their carbs down that steeply, it wouldn't have much impact on their hunger. Because even when they were eating that 100 gram meal, their blood sugars weren't rising high enough to trigger a strong hunger response. They don't have to cut down on carbs to get rid of the gnawing physiological hunger that makes so many other people overeat, because, as a truly normal person, they never experience it. That's why people with truly normal blood sugars who need to lose weight can succeed on any diet that cuts down on their calorie intake, including diets very high in carbohydrate like conventional low fat and vegan diets.

You might ask at this point, why a normal person would ever need to diet at all, if blood sugar-related hunger is such a major cause of weight gain. The answer is simple: Even though they aren't driven by relentless hunger, normal people still eat too much.

Everyone, no matter how normal their blood sugar, will gain weight when they eat more calories each day than they burn. And because we live in an environment where extremely high calorie food is constantly thrust beneath our noses that's not hard to do.

Normal people may not be driven to eat by hunger, but they overeat because there are free donuts in the break room, or because they're served a muffin the size of a small loaf of bread at the local coffee shop and eat it all. They gain weight because their Aunt Fanny won't rest until they have another serving of her famous pecan pie, because eating is something they do when they're sad, or because their TVs display endless shrimp, along with endless pizza, chips, and pasta.

If you'll remember, normal people start secreting insulin when they *see* food, in the expectation that they will soon be eating it. Our genes haven't yet caught up to the idea that TV can show us realistic-looking food we aren't actually going to eat.

But when a normal person who isn't driven to eat by a raging physiological hunger signal starts paying attention, they can usually cut down on their portion sizes and eliminate the excess foods they have been eating out of habit. And when they do, their weight starts to drop very quickly.

Cutting Carbs when Blood Sugar Is Not Normal

Something very different happens when a person whose blood sugar is *not* truly normal cuts down on their carbs.

The reason their blood sugar is higher than normal is almost always because their insulin is not able to do its job. When their blood sugar rises towards 120 mg/dl some people's pancreases may fail to secrete enough insulin to take care of the incoming glucose. This is very typical of people who have inherited one of many known genes associated with Type 2 diabetes.

Others may have pancreases that secrete the usual amount of insulin, but because insulin receptors inside their cells have stopped responding properly to insulin their insulin is ineffective. Sometimes the reason these receptors have stopped responding is because their muscle cells don't burn glucose properly. So to keep from getting flooded with glucose they can't use, cells in their muscles and liver start to ignore insulin. When that happens we call them *insulin resistant*.

Other people have livers that have become deaf to insulin's signaling because they have become clogged with fat. Normal livers dump glucose into the bloodstream during periods when we are fasting to keep our blood sugars from dropping dangerously low. But when insulin levels rise, a healthy liver takes that as a signal to stop dumping glucose.

Insulin resistant livers fail to respond to rising insulin levels. So they dump glucose into the bloodstream even at meal times, ignoring the fact that blood sugar is already rising because glucose is coming in from digested food. This pushes blood sugars into the range above normal after every meal.

Whatever the reason why your insulin isn't getting the job done, if your blood sugar is rising over that truly normal 120 mg/dl level, the single most effective way of lowering it — far more effective than any medication on the market or even exercise — is to cut back on your intake of carbohydrates.

That's because when insulin is struggling to lower your blood sugar, every added gram you eat over the amount your insulin can process raises your blood sugar 2.5 to 5 mg/dl depending on your weight. (The heavier you are, the less a gram of carbohydrate will raise your blood sugar.) It follows, then, that every gram of carbohydrate you *don't* eat when your insulin is struggling will lower your blood sugar by that same 2.5 to 5 mg/dl.

That said, we can't show you a graph of how someone with an abnormal glucose tolerance would respond to cutting out 25 or 45 grams of carbohydrate from a single meal, because how much carbohydrate each abnormal person's body can handle is so different. Some people will see a completely normal pattern after removing the bun from their hamburger. Others may have to cut out the bun and the fries. Still others will have to ditch the bun, the fries, and milk. That's why when we discuss how to customize your own low carb diet in Chapter 9, we will put such emphasis on the importance of learning just how much carbohydrate your own body can tolerate.

High Blood Sugars Cause Secondary Insulin Resistance

There's another factor to consider before we leave this topic. If your blood sugars spike very high after you eat high carbohydrate meals, the more you lower your blood sugars by cutting out carbohydrates, the easier it gets to lower them further. That's because, as you lower how high your blood sugars peak, you also eliminate something called *secondary insulin resistance*. This effect is illustrated in Figure 5, where you can see the sharp drop in their post-meal blood sugars that occurs in a hypothetical individual after their blood sugar peaks drop below 180 mg/dl. (Ferrannini, 1992).

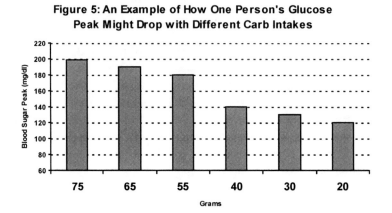

Figure 5: An Example of How One Person's Glucose Peak Might Drop with Different Carb Intakes

Secondary insulin resistance is called "secondary" to differentiate it from your underlying, genetically-determined level of insulin resistance, which is largely determined by factors like how efficiently your cells burn glucose. Secondary insulin resistance is not something you are born with or something you have to live with. It's extra insulin resistance that only kicks in when your blood sugars rise to abnormal heights.

Secondary insulin resistance is your body's way of protecting your cells from the damage they might experience from having insulin push an overwhelming influx of glucose into the cell all at once. It becomes a factor after your blood sugar rises over some threshold—for many people it's somewhere around 180 mg/dl. Most importantly, secondary insulin resistance makes you more insulin resistant, no matter what your inborn level of insulin resistance might be.

The good news here is that this secondary insulin resistance goes away as soon as you keep your blood sugars from rising over 140 mg/dl, which is one reason why cutting carbs can make such a big difference in people's blood sugars especially after they have become prediabetic. As soon as you cut your carbs down to the level where they no longer push your blood sugars up to that 180 mg/dl threshold, you stop experiencing secondary insulin resistance and your insulin works more efficiently. Now the same amount of insulin can process much more carbohydrate than it could when your blood sugars were higher.[6]

Eliminating secondary insulin resistance will also help ratchet down your feelings of hunger. This is because the more insulin sensitive you are, the more likely you are to secrete several hormones that reduce hunger, a topic we'll explore more fully in Chapter 5. (Stock, 2005)

Everyone's blood sugar will drop at a different rate when they cut carbohydrates out of their meals, but it's important to note that, contrary to what you may have been told, how fast your blood sugar normalizes has nothing to do with your weight.

Weight loss does not normalize blood sugars. Eating less carbs at mealtimes normalizes blood sugars—even if you don't lose a single pound. In fact, often people who are of normal weight or only slightly overweight who have abnormally high blood sugars will see *less* of a drop in their blood sugar when they cut their carbs than do people who are very heavy. That's because thin people who develop abnormally high blood sugars often do so because they aren't secreting enough insulin. When insulin isn't being secreted properly, even low carb meals may raise blood sugars quite high.[7]

But whatever the underlying reason for high blood sugars, people who have them almost always find that when they lower their carbohydrate intake enough to flatten out their blood sugar they stop feeling hungry and start to lose weight—sometimes without any conscious attempt to diet.

Mind you, there's no miracle cure here. Once you turn off that hunger signal, you still have to cut back on your eating to lose weight—just like the normal people we discussed earlier. You'll have to become more conscious of what you're eating and eat less. But once your brain isn't sending out hunger signals in response to quickly dropping blood sugars, you'll find this a lot easier to do.

---

[6] High levels of fat circulating in the bloodstream—triglycerides—also cause secondary insulin resistance, which is why many doctors erroneously believe that eating fat will make your blood sugars go up. In fact, eating carbohydrates is what mainly raises your triglycerides, and lowering your carbohydrate intake will cause your triglyceride levels to drop fairly quickly, contributing to the drop in secondary insulin resistance. Concentrations of fat within your cells, which we'll discuss later on, also contribute to insulin resistance, but they may derive from problems within the cell that aren't solved by weight loss.

[7] Some heavy people also develop high blood sugars because they aren't secreting normal amounts of insulin. This usually happens when they are suffering an autoimmune attack. When this happens, eventually their blood sugars may become dangerously high. If your blood sugar doesn't normalize when you cut your carbs and continues to worsen, you should see a doctor and get tested for autoimmune diabetes.

At this point it might strike you that if the low carb diet exerts its primary effects by normalizing blood sugars, many people whose blood sugars are only slightly abnormal may get all the benefits of a low carb diet from eating *any* diet that normalizes their blood sugar, even if it is a lot higher in carbs than the low carb diets described in bestselling low carb diet books, and this is indeed the case.

Most people, including many whose blood sugars are only mildly abnormal, will lose weight and greatly improve their health as soon as they cut their carbohydrates just enough to achieve a truly normal blood sugar pattern that doesn't trigger the brain's fear that they will run out of vital glucose.

People who keep their blood sugars under 120 mg/dl at all times see their cholesterol levels and blood pressure drop. Their A1Cs also drop to the level that corresponds to a very low risk of heart attack. If they have been diagnosed with diabetes, they don't develop new diabetic complications no matter how high their blood sugars might have been in the past. Best of all, with the hunger signal stilled, they find that losing weight, while never easy, becomes a matter of learning how to eat more mindfully and reducing their food intake so that they eat less than they burn each day. [8]

What Happens When You Cut *Way* Down on Carbs

Not everyone will normalize their blood sugar by substituting a salad for fries when they order a hamburger. Some people's blood sugars stay higher than normal after modest carb restriction, especially people whose blood sugars rise well into the prediabetic range. This may be because their beta cells don't secrete insulin properly or because they have such severe primary insulin resistance that even huge amounts of insulin can no longer normalize their blood sugars.

Whatever the cause, if you fall into this category, the only way you may be able to drop your blood sugar into the normal range and avoid those hunger-provoking plunges is to drop your carbohydrate intake below 12 grams per meal, but as soon as you do that, a whole new

---

[8] People who have been diabetic for a long time may have established complications which will seem to worsen as they normalize their blood sugar. For example, people who have damaged retinas caused by years of exposure to high blood sugars may experience a temporary worsening of this retinal damage as toxic compounds previously introduced by high blood sugars exit the eye. Even so, long-term studies have shown their vision is far better years later than that of people who had the same high blood sugars who did *not* lower their blood sugars. By the same token, people with nerve damage may experience nerve pain after normalizing their blood sugars. This is caused by numb, dead nerves regenerating because blood flow improves when blood sugar levels are normal. As the nerves continue to heal, the pain should stop.

suite of physiological changes will take place in your body—changes which cause the most misunderstood effects of the low carbohydrate diet.

Within a few days of dropping your carbohydrate intake to an extremely low level you'll experience an immediate and dramatic loss of weight. You'll not only see it on the scale, you'll feel it. Your arms and legs will feel slimmer. Your abdomen will shrink. When this happens, if you are like most people, you'll conclude that the low carb diet is indeed a miraculous diet for weight loss. Having already lost ten or fifteen pounds in a few weeks, you'll thrill to the thought that you can look forward to losing 40, 50, or even 100 pounds in only another few months. In fact, this isn't likely to happen, even though the bestselling low carb diet books make it sound like it's common. In fact, this early, fast, weight loss stops fairly quickly, and after it does, weight loss proceeds at a much slower pace.

The authors of these books also don't mention that the weight you lose so quickly during the first few weeks of the diet comes back immediately as soon as you eat more than 100 grams of carb in a single day. It's possible they neglect to explain this rapid initial weight loss and instant regain because they believe that it motivates people to stick to their diets. If so, they're entitled to their beliefs. But it's my belief, after years of observing hundreds of people eating very low carb diets, that the lack of frankness about what causes this speedy weight loss and equally speedy regain is a major reason why so many once-enthusiastic low carb dieters not only give up their diets, but do so in a way that leads them to catastrophic weight regain.

The truth is that the highly motivating quick weight loss and the devastating instant regain that occur on a very low carb diet have nothing to do with getting rid of the excess fat you're carrying on your body. It's all about what happens to your glycogen stores—the same glycogen stores discussed in the previous chapter, which hold the emergency glucose you use when you aren't eating enough carbohydrate to supply your brain's constant demand for glucose.

What a Very Low Carb Diet Does to Glycogen

We talked earlier about how glycogen is the starchy substance your liver creates to store glucose for immediate use any time you haven't recently eaten any sugary or starchy foods. We also mentioned that scientists estimate that your liver stores enough glycogen to supply the amount of glucose your brain burns through in a day.

When you eat so little starch and sugar that your meals no longer supply the glucose your brain needs, your liver draws more heavily on its stored glycogen and converts it back to glucose. You can tell when this starts to happen because when you burn a lot of glycogen, you start having to urinate far more than normal.

This occurs because glycogen molecules attract water molecules that bond to them. The exact amount of water stored is estimated to be roughly 4 grams of water for every gram of glycogen. (Eaton, 1934) When those glycogen molecules are broken down into their component glucose molecules, the water that was bonded to them is released and excreted by your kidneys.

When this happens, your body will also dump a significant amount of sodium and potassium. One study found that when dieters embark on a very low carb diet they excrete higher than normal amounts of sodium for 7 days. Their potassium excretion is higher than normal for up to 14 days, after which it stabilizes. This loss of potassium can cause muscle cramping. (Rabast, 1981) This loss of sodium and potassium may further increase your water loss as well as reducing your blood pressure.

So it makes sense that the first weight you lose as you deplete your stored glycogen is the weight of the burned glycogen and all the water that was bonded to it. Because four grams of water are bound to every molecule of glycogen, that lost water will be four times as heavy as the lost glycogen.

The textbooks tell us that people have no more than 150 grams of glycogen stored in their livers, 95% of which can be fully depleted. If this were true, when you burned off your glycogen you'd get rid of, at most, 143 grams of glycogen which would release another 570 grams of water. This should result in a total weight loss of roughly 713 grams or 1.6 pounds.

The textbooks also tell us that the average person carries another 350 grams of glycogen which is stored in their muscles. Not all of that glycogen will be depleted when you cut way down on your dietary carbs, since only prolonged and vigorous exercise will fully deplete muscle glycogen.

Even when your muscles have depleted their glycogen stores, they are able to partially refill them even if you haven't eaten more carbohydrate. They do this by recycling the lactic acid that is produced by the anaerobic form of respiration our muscles use during high intensity exercise. It is estimated that one third of muscle glycogen remains, even in people eating very low carb diets. (McDonald, 1998, p. 121) The weight of the two thirds of your muscle glycogen you can burn off and of its associated water would account for another 2.5 pounds of the weight you lose over the first few days of a very low carb diet. (Bergstrom, 1967, cited by McDonald, op. cit.)

All in all, the textbook descriptions of glycogen suggest that the first 4.1 lbs you lose on a low carb diet can be completely explained by the loss of your liver and muscle glycogen.

Because glycogen is estimated to make up as much as 8% of your liver's weight, burning through it makes a noticeable reduction in the size of your liver. Since your liver is situated in your abdomen just above your waist, when it shrinks your midriff shrinks with it, providing an immediate loss of what chirpy gym salespeople like to call "inches." With your liver shrunk, you feel instantly thinner, which is highly motivating. Your muscles' loss of glycogen may also make your thighs and upper arms shrink, too. But as good as it feels, you haven't yet lost any fat.

Do Some People Store Abnormal Amounts of Glycogen?

Critics of the diet often argue that most of the weight loss achieved by very low carb diets is due *only* to this loss of glycogen and water. Advocates of the diet retort that after you lose the 4 lbs attributable to glycogen the rest of the weight you lose will come from burning fat.

I used to believe this, too, until I noticed how common it was for dieters participating in online discussion groups to lose as much as 20 pounds during the first month of their very low carb diets, only to stall out completely after that. The same thing happened to me. I lost 20 lbs within a little more than a month, followed by a complete stall that continued for several years.

As I saw more people reporting this same phenomenon, I began to wonder if perhaps people with abnormal glucose metabolisms might store a lot *more* glycogen than the average cited in textbooks. If that were true, much more of the weight they lost so quickly during those early weeks might be due to the loss of their larger than usual glycogen stores and all the water that had been bonded to them.

A bit of hunting through musty old research papers confirmed this was very possible, because it turns out that these glycogen estimates come from two kinds of research: research conducted in rats and research conducted in young, healthy male college students.

Rats turn out to have a glucose metabolism that varies from that of humans in several small but significant ways. For example, the insulin-producing cells in the rat pancreas respond differently than do human beta cells to *ketones,* which are important chemicals produced when our muscle cells start burning fat instead of glucose, (Macdonald, 2011) The young male college students who figured in the human research, most of it conducted in the 1950s and '60s, were far slimmer and fitter than people embarking on low carb diets today. This made it more likely that someone who wasn't a rodent or a thin, fit man in their 20s might store a lot more glycogen than those averages suggest.

There's evidence this is true. Some of it comes from a study where twelve women whose weights ranged from 143 to 238 pounds were first put on the identical standard (i.e. high carbohydrate) diet for eleven days to eliminate any effects on their glycogen caused by the diet they'd been eating before the study started. At the end of this cleanout period, the women were put on a very low carbohydrate diet that provided only 1,700 calories a day.

Their glycogen stores were estimated before and after four days of eating the very low carbohydrate diet using a sophisticated technique that relies on the fact that potassium is associated with glycogen in a known ratio. This allowed the researchers to use a measurement of the women's whole body potassium to estimate their glycogen stores.

What is delightful about this study is that instead of providing the data in the usual way, which it to report only the *average* value for the group, the researchers in this study published the data for all twelve participants, including their starting and ending weights, as well as the amount of their weight loss over the first four days of the very low carbohydrate diet that was attributed to their loss of glycogen.

The amounts of glycogen these individual dieters lost varied greatly from person to person. One 236 lb dieter who lost about 15 lbs over four days appeared to have lost only 80 grams of glycogen, which is less than 3 ounces. Another dieter who started out at 186 lbs and lost 9 lbs was estimated to have lost 1,066 grams of glycogen, 2.30 lbs, which, when you add in the water associated with it would account for roughly 10 pounds of glycogen and be enough to account for every pound of the weight this dieter had lost over those first few days.

You can see the whole table of weight and glycogen losses in the journal article, "Glycogen storage: illusions of easy weight loss, excessive weight regain, and distortions in estimates of body composition," (Kreitzman, 1992) which you'll find at:

http://www.ajcn.org/content/56/1/292S.long

Even if the methodology that was used to estimate glycogen stores in this study is not entirely accurate, it certainly suggests that there is much wider variation in how much glycogen individuals may be storing than is usually reported. In addition, it makes it clear that the amount of glycogen stored doesn't necessarily correlate to the person's weight.

Insight into *why* a person might be storing a much larger amount of glycogen than expected comes from another study where normal, healthy young men were fed a single meal containing a whopping 479 grams of carbohydrate—which because they were, in fact, normal, raised their blood sugars to an average peak of only 119 mg/dl.

The scientists analyzed the young men's breath with a respirometer to determine how much glucose and fat they had burned over the hours after they had consumed this carb-up. They estimated from these measurements that these young men had each added, on average, another 346 grams of glycogen to their pre-existing glycogen stores. That's 1 lb 5 oz of new glycogen from just one extremely high carb meal. This led the researchers to conclude, "The capacity for glycogen storage in man is larger than generally believed." (Acheson, 1982)

If people with completely normal glucose metabolisms can pack on that much extra glycogen after a single carbfest, how much could a person pack on over the years if they had an abnormal glucose metabolism that made them hungry enough to eat high carb meals like that every day?

I can't find human research that would answer that question conclusively, but rat research suggests that the amount of glycogen stored in the liver might go *way* up in people with only slightly abnormal blood sugars. Rats whose blood sugar was maintained at an average level of 108 mg/dl for 3 hours, stored 2.6 times as much glycogen in their livers as did normal rats. And when those rats' blood sugar was kept at 180 mg/dl for those 3 hours—the level that people with prediabetes reach every day—the amount of glycogen they stored rose to almost 4 *times* normal. The study concludes, "The results confirm that blood glucose concentration is the major short-term regulator of glycogen synthase activity in the liver." (Kruszynska, 1986)

There's something else you eat that turns into glycogen: fructose. Fructose is another simple sugar that when bonded to glucose turns into sucrose. It's also found in high concentrations in high fructose corn syrup (HFCS). Though you will usually read that HFCS is only 55% fructose, it's been detected at concentrations up to 65% by researchers who analyzed "popular sugar-sweetened beverages" in the lab. (Ventura, 2011)

The fructose you eat doesn't turn directly into blood glucose—which is why if you eat pure fructose it won't raise your blood sugar after meals. But over time the liver converts dietary fructose into either fat or glycogen. Some research in humans shows that infusions of fructose raise the amount of glycogen stored in the liver 3.6 times more than do infusions of dietary glucose. This suggests that heavy consumption of sugar or high fructose corn syrup might also explain why some people are carrying many more pounds of glycogen than others. (Nilsson, 1974)

All this suggests that a person whose blood sugar is slightly abnormal and who has been eating a lot of sugary, processed foods and drinking sodas full of HFCS could accumulate extremely large stores of glycogen that would take not days, but weeks to burn off. From that it also follows that much, if not all, of the weight dieters lose during the early weeks or even, in extreme cases, months of a very low carb diet may, in fact, be due to the loss of this glycogen and its associated supply of water, especially in the case of dieters whose weight loss halts abruptly after losing these quick first pounds.

Quick Weight Loss, Devastating Regain

The downside of the quick weight loss attributable to glycogen is that this weight comes back on as soon as you eat enough sugar or starch to allow your liver and muscles to rebuild their glycogen stores. This can happen after a single meal, because it only takes eating more than 70 to 110 grams of carbohydrates to trigger this process. The exact amount depends on your size.

The day you consume more than this amount of carbohydrate, your glycogen stores start to fill up, and when they do that they also bind four times their weight in water. That's why consuming a single off-plan meal will typically cause a low carb dieter to pack on as much as 2 lbs immediately. If you keep on eating carbohydrate-rich meals, every bit of weight you lost that could be attributed to glycogen will return. If you were someone with a lot of stored glycogen on board, this may be a surprising amount of weight.

And you don't just end up with the same glycogen-associated weight you started out with. Remember how we said earlier that protecting the brain's precious glucose supply is Job One? Well, a bout of glycogen depletion is interpreted by your brain as being an episode of starvation. That causes some changes in your hormones that ensure that not only do you *refill* your glycogen stores, but that you *expand* them so that the *next* time you find yourself in an environment short on nourishing carbohydrates your brain has a *bigger* store of glycogen to draw on.

One study found that after a carbohydrate refeeding that followed glycogen depletion, the amount of muscle glycogen stored rose to more than *twice* normal. (Begstrom, op. cit.). A similar effect was found in liver glycogen. When humans were fasted and then fed a very low carbohydrate diet that depleted their liver glycogen, high carbohydrate refeeding increased their liver glycogen, as measured via needle biopsies, to what the researchers called, "supernormal values." These were almost double what they had been at the start of the experiment. (Nilsson, 1973)

This short-term response to glycogen deprivation should wane over time after a person has adapted to the fully fed state. Many people who have lost weight successfully on very low carb diets do maintain their weight losses while eating at a level high enough to refill their glycogen, and their glycogen levels appear to drop back eventually to their original pre-diet level.

The Shift into a Ketogenic State

Once days or weeks of eating a very low carb diet have depleted your liver's store of glycogen, glucose becomes a precious and carefully hoarded resource. All the body's cells that are able to burn fats switch to burning fat exclusively, to preserve what glucose is available for those critical neurons in the brain that require it.

One byproduct of the process by which cells burn fat is a chemical called a ketone body or *ketone.* As your cells continue to burn fat, the concentration of ketones they give off starts to rise in the bloodstream. A diet that causes high levels of ketones to be produced is called a *ketogenic diet.*

Ketones have a bad reputation in the medical world, because when the concentration of ketones in the bloodstream becomes extremely high, they acidify the blood and cause a very dangerous condition called ketoacidosis, which can be fatal.

Ketoacidosis rarely occurs except in people with Type 1 diabetes who may experience it when their blood sugars go extremely high— for example over 500 mg/dl. Ketoacidosis also occurs in people suffering from kidney failure, extreme dehydration, liver failure, cancer, or poisoning. In these conditions, the normal mechanisms the body usually uses to get rid of excess ketones break down, and the ketone levels rise to damaging heights. (NIH: Ketones)

But despite their association with this dangerous condition, ketones are a normal part of our blood chemistry. They are produced whenever our cells switch to burning fat instead of glucose. This happens any time we have gone more than 4 hours without eating, for example, at night while we are sleeping.

When a person with normal blood sugars and healthy organs experiences a rise in the level of ketones in their blood, their bodies eliminate these ketones via their urine, and, if the ketone level is very high, in their breath—which gives a characteristic, banana-y smell to some, but fortunately not all, dieters who eat ketogenic diets.

Since ketones don't appear in the urine until the body is burning significant amounts of fat, some low carb dieters test their urine with the ketone test strips available at the drugstore to verify that they are, in fact, burning fat instead of glucose in most of their tissues. Some of the better studies conducted with low carb dieters also measure their subject's ketone levels, in order to verify that the dieters are really eating a very low carb diet.

The Critical Role of Protein in a Ketogenic Diet

Once the liver's glycogen stores are gone, where do those vital cells in the brain that can't burn fat get the glucose they need? The answer is, largely, *from protein.*

Like carbohydrates and fats, proteins are made out of carbon, hydrogen, and oxygen, but they differ from these two other macronutrients in that proteins also contain significant amounts of nitrogen.

When we eat proteins, digestion disassembles them into the amino acids out of which they were made, which then travel through the bloodstream. These amino acids are absorbed by cells that use them to repair damaged DNA, grow new cells, and build the many hormones, enzymes, lipids, neurotransmitters, and immune system components that keep your body functioning.

Unlike carbohydrate and fat, your body cannot store excess protein. When proteins are digested, they break down into amino acids and circulate in the bloodstream, so cells can pick them up and synthesize them into useful proteins. The liver and kidneys dispose of any excess amino acids by converting them into glucose through the process called gluconeogenesis. They do this by first extracting the nitrogen from the amino acids and converting it into ammonia. This ammonia is then converted into urea, which is excreted in the urine. Once the nitrogen is disposed of, the carbon, hydrogen, and oxygen that are left over from the amino acids are converted into glucose, which can then be stored as glycogen.

The glucose produced from protein through this process is what keeps your brain ticking when you're in a glycogen-depleted state. Thanks to gluconeogenesis, up to 58% of the excess protein you consume can be converted into glucose. If protein is very scarce, the liver can also extract a very small amount of glucose from fat. But when protein is very scarce, mostly what happens is that the liver will synthesize the glucose it needs by breaking down proteins extracted from the body's own muscle tissue. This is dangerous because one of the tissues that will be cannibalized to create this precious glucose is the heart muscle.

It is because the very low carbohydrate diet requires that you eat enough extra protein to supply your brain with glucose that low carb diets are often promoted as "high protein" diets. But the emphasis diet book authors have put on the idea that the ketogenic diet is a high protein diet is misleading, because after the first few weeks on a ketogenic diet the actual amount of extra protein you need to provide your brain with its glucose is very modest.

That's because, though it is true that your brain needs about 100 grams of glucose a day when you start out on your ketogenic diet, this changes once your muscle cells have all switched to burning fat. As you'll recall, ketones are a byproduct of burning fat, and unlike fats, ketones can cross the blood-brain barrier. Once they do, your neurons can burn these ketones to provide some, though not all, of their energy needs. So once you have enough ketones in your blood, your brain's requirement for glucose drops to only about 40 grams a day. (McDonald, 1998, p. 45)

Since only 58% of protein can be converted into glucose, it would take 69 grams of extra protein to provide this additional 40 grams of glucose for your brain. You could get that by eating an additional 11.5 ounces of a high protein food like meat, fish, or hard cheese, since these high protein foods contain 6 grams of protein per ounce.

But this calculation assumes that you are consuming no carbohydrate at all, which unless you are living entirely on muscle meat, isn't likely. There are trace amounts of carbohydrate in many foods you might not think contain them, like coffee, eggs, and many cheeses. Even if you were eating only 20 grams of carbohydrate a day, once your brain started burning ketones, you would only need to eat an additional 5 ounces of high protein food to supply the protein out of which the liver will make that glucose needed for your brain.

With every additional ten grams of carbohydrate you eat, you need one less ounce of high protein food. So by the time you are eating 70 grams of carbohydrate each day you won't need to consume any additional protein to supply glucose for your brain.

You will, of course, *also* need to keep eating enough protein to repair your muscles and furnish your cells with the raw materials for the protein-based components they synthesize. The formula commonly used to estimate how much protein this requires tells you to eat .8

grams of protein for every kilogram of your total body weight. A kilogram is 2.2 pounds. So a person weighing 150 lbs (68 kg) would need to eat 54 grams of protein for body maintenance, in addition to any extra protein needed to generate glucose. They could get that 54 grams by eating 9 ounces of high protein food like meat or eggs. A 300 pounder would need to consume double that amount. If you are doing hard physical labor or intensive body building you will also need more. But the average dieter who, at best, spends an hour at the gym a few times a week will not.

Eating more protein than is needed to repair and replace tissues and supply extra glucose is not particularly healthy. Eating protein requires your body to secrete insulin and if your insulin isn't working well, eating a lot of protein which turns into glucose via gluconeogenesis can raise your blood sugar. Because the process of gluconeogenesis also raises the concentration of urea in your urine, it can cause that urine to become corrosive and lead to rashes. Eating too much protein also contributes to the bad breath associated with the ketogenic diet because some of the excess ammonia compounds that result from the breakdown of protein are excreted via the breath.

Burning Fat on a Ketogenic Diet

Bestselling low carb diet books often suggest that once you have shifted your body into a ketogenic state and turned your body into a fat burning machine, rapid weight loss is bound to follow.

This ignores the fact that while your cells are certainly burning a lot of fat on a very low carb diet, the first fat they burn through is the *dietary* fat you eat. Since the very low carb diet is typically very high in fat—the usual percentage of fat in medically-recommended very low carb diets approaches 60%—it's very easy to eat a ketogenic diet that provides all the fat your cells will burn through the day.

The thousands of dieters who show up asking on low carb diet discussion boards how it could be that their weight loss has stalled so completely when they are turning ketone test strips dark purple every day verifies that this is not an infrequent occurrence.

There is little evidence that being in a ketogenic state, in and of itself, turbocharges weight loss for most people. Nor is there any physiological reason why it should. Some low carb enthusiasts claim that excess calories are lost when we excrete those urinary ketones. But though the ketones excreted in your urine do represent some lost calories, the actual amount of calories excreted in the form of ketones is very small, ranging between 40 and 90 calories a day. (McDonald, 1998, p. 33)

Others argue that there is a slight advantage to ketogenic diets that comes from something called the "Thermic effect of protein." (Halton, 2004) This argument stems from the fact that it takes more cellular energy to digest protein than it does to digest carbohydrate—about 20-35% as opposed to 5-15% for carbs. So a diet that is higher in protein than the standard mixed diet may be using up more calories in digesting that excess protein. However, the quality of the studies used to defend this theory is poor and uncontrolled for too many variables. Besides, as was previously mentioned, a properly constituted very low carb diet should not be extremely high in protein.

As you will see when we turn to the research studies in the next chapter, there is little evidence that very low carb diets produce more weight loss than other diets that supply the same number of calories. To get rid of fat you must still eat less calories than you burn, no matter what diet you're eating. Burn 3,500 calories more than you eat and you'll lose a single pound of body fat.

Given the weakness of data supporting any other explanation for how a low carb diet might speed up weight loss, it's most likely that the real advantage that dieters get from being in a ketogenic state is that it abolishes hunger and makes it easier to cut down dramatically on food intake, which *will* cause weight loss. This is likely, given how many people post on low carb discussion boards that they forget to eat when they are in a fully ketogenic state. But whether the diet abolishes hunger by flattening their blood sugars or whether high concentration of ketones in the blood have a hunger-damping effect on the brain is unknown.

Arguing against the idea that ketones have a magical effect on hunger is the fact that ketone levels can be very high in people who are starving, since their bodies burn through their body fat stores in the absence of dietary fat. But people who are actually starving become obsessed with food to the point where thoughts of food completely take over their lives.

The Beginner's Luck Syndrome

There is one interesting anecdotal effect associated with ketogenic diets, the so-called "beginner's luck" phenomenon. I have not been able to find it documented in any research, but it is often reported by people who post on the web, so it may very well be a real phenomenon, though perhaps one that is relatively rare.

The beginner's luck syndrome occurs when someone embarks on their very first very low carb diet and experiences speedy, dramatic weight loss that continues long enough and results in a weight loss large enough that this loss cannot be due solely to glycogen depletion. The lucky people who experience this will lose as much as 100 pounds very quickly—sometimes within six months of starting their first very low carb diet. From what I've observed online, it seems like the people who experience beginner's luck are almost always males.

However, there's a reason this phenomenon is called "beginner's luck." Because if these people go off their low carb diet, return to their old eating habits, regain their lost weight, and attempt to take it off a second time with the same low carb diet, they will often find that their weight loss this second time proceeds far more slowly. If they are patient and persistent they can be just as successful this second time, but their weight loss is likely to take longer.

I have no idea what causes this or even if it is a real phenomenon. But because it's reported often enough online that it's possible that it is real, if you are fortunate enough to experience beginner's luck and drop a lot of weight very quickly, don't be lured into thinking that you don't have to be vigilant in maintaining that weight loss, because doing it again will be much harder and take a lot longer.

Points to Remember from This Chapter:

1. The worse your blood sugar is, the more impact cutting carbs will make.

2. Only by testing after meals can you determine how many grams of carbohydrate you can eat at a meal without pushing your blood sugar out of the normal range.

3. Eating a ketogenic diet drains the body's glycogen stores and may produce surprisingly large weight losses and frighteningly swift weight gains due entirely to glycogen depletion.

4. There is evidence that some people store far more glycogen than normal, especially those with slightly abnormal blood sugars and those who consume a lot of sugar and HFCS. Depleting your glycogen by eating a low carb diet is likely to mean you end up storing a lot more glycogen when you carb up again.

5. Ketogenic dieters do burn fat for energy but they burn dietary fat before they burn body fat unless there is a caloric deficit.

6. Though ketogenic dieters do need to eat extra protein to supply the brain's glucose needs the actual amount needed is not that large. Too much protein turns into glucose and may raise blood sugar and insulin levels.

Chapter 3
How Low Carb Diets Compare to Others

Back when I started eating a low carb diet in the late 1990s, doctors and nutritionists universally warned that the low carb diet was dangerous. Eating all that fat would worsen our cholesterol. Eating all that protein would damage our kidneys. The authors of bestselling low carb diet books like *Dr. Atkins' New Diet Revolution, Protein Power,* and *Dr. Bernstein's Diabetes Solution* assured us this wasn't true, though they often supported their claims with little more than logical arguments and stories about the wonderful results their patients had experienced. Some cited a few cherry-picked studies to prove the safety and efficacy of the low carb diet, but those studies were inaccessible to their readers in those pre-Google days, so it was hard to know if they really proved what the authors said they did.

Because of the relentless attacks launched by opponents of the low carb diet, the authors of low carb diet books took a strident, evangelical tone that cast scorn on their opponent's claims. That same tone was adopted by many of us who tried low carb diets and found them to be effective. But over the years, though I repeated to others the arguments I'd read in the diet books, I started wondering how true they really were.

I started my diabetes research because I questioned the validity of the claims Dr. Bernstein made in his landmark *Diabetes Solution* book that normal people's blood sugars were always 83 mg/dl and that raising blood sugars only slightly above this level would cause diabetic complications.

Dr. Bernstein insisted that people with diabetes had no choice but to eat a ketogenic diet, which many of us found to be very burdensome. When I delved into the research I found that his main argument was true — lowering carbohydrates is the single most powerful tool we have for normalizing blood sugar and normalizing blood sugars will prevent diabetic complications. But the research did not back up his claim that normal people's blood sugars were always under 100 mg/dl. In fact, a lot of studies suggested that the level at which complications began to appear was considerably higher than what he'd told us.

I documented my findings on my Blood Sugar 101 web page (http://bloodsugar101.com). Since then, I have heard from many people who were not able to adhere to Dr. Bernstein's extremely low carb diet for more than a year or two, but who *were* able to succeed eating a nonketogenic diet that provided slightly more carbohydrate each day. That diets still controlled their blood sugars, prevented complications, and was much easier to stick to.

So when I decided to write this book about the benefits of the low carb diet for people whose blood sugar issues were far milder than those of us with diabetes, I found myself wondering if the ketogenic diet recommended by so many bestselling diet books for weight loss was similarly oversold.

To answer that question, I took a fresh look at what high quality, peer-reviewed research had to say about the claims made by the authors of bestselling low carb diet books. I knew from looking into this topic a decade ago, that, back when most of the groundbreaking low carb diet books had been published in the 1990s, studies had made it look as if low carb diets were less healthy than the low fat diets that had come into fashion in the 1980s.

But I also remembered that the "low carbohydrate" diets discussed in those studies were almost always diets that, while they *were* lower in carbohydrate than the typical diet of that time, which was 60% carbohydrate, were still quite high in carbs. Most of them got at least 40% of their calories from carbohydrate. That worked out to 150 to 200 grams a day, which was far more than the 20-100 grams a day that the low carb books of the 1990s recommended.

These older studies certainly confirmed that diets that got 40% of their calories from carbohydrate did not outperform other diets, and that when these moderate carb diets were also high in fat, they did, in fact, appear to worsen cholesterol profiles.

Since then a lot of research into the effects of truly low carb diets has been published. The low carb diet fad that peaked around 2000 sparked renewed interest in the topic among nutritionists, and after the death of Dr. Robert Atkins in 2003, an infusion of money from the Atkins Foundation became available to fund quite a few smaller academic and medical studies, too. So there now are high quality studies from which we can draw conclusions about the real impact of eating a truly low carb diet.

Most of the recent, large, well-funded studies that tested Atkins-style diets have been published in high impact journals. Because of how controversial their findings were, their results were the medical equivalent of "man bites dog." They made it onto the nightly news and into morning papers because they reported, much to everyone's surprise, that what everyone thought was a "heart attack on a plate" diet, where people gorged on fat, turned out to pose no threat to heart health. Not only that, but some of the new studies found that the Atkins-style diets, produced better weight loss and healthier cholesterol profiles than the low fat diets recommended by the American Diabetes Association and the American Heart Association.

I'd known this, because these studies had been hailed as a breakthrough by many of my friends in the online diet community and we all avidly followed the media reports. But when I went back and dug into the full texts of these studies, which were now available online for free, as they had not been when they were newly published, I found they contained other, more interesting findings. These findings had not been covered by the press and are, therefore, unknown to many of the low carb enthusiasts who have pointed for years to these published studies as evidence that the diet is healthy and effective.

We'll start out by looking at the biggest studies, the ones that made it into your newspapers and onto TV. These were all large studies where groups of people eating a very low carb diet, almost always in the form prescribed by Atkins, were pitted against groups of people eating other popular diets.

The Tufts Study

The first large-scale study comparing a very low carb diet to other diets was "Comparison of the Atkins, Ornish, Weight Watchers, and Zone Diets for Weight Loss and Heart Disease Risk Reduction" which was published in 2005 in the *Journal of the American Medical Association* by a team of researchers from Tufts-New England Medical Center. This study got a lot of play in the media as it was the first study to make it clear how wrong the many mainstream critics of the low carb diet had been when they claimed it was harmful. (Dansinger, 2005)

This study followed 160 participants, half men and half women, whose average weight was 220 lbs, and whose average age was 47. Some were diabetic. They were randomly assigned to either the Atkins diet, the Zone diet—which prescribes 40% carbs, 30% protein, and 30% fat, the Weight Watchers calorie-restricted diet, or the Ornish very low fat diet that prescribes 75% carbs, 15% protein, and 10% fat. After 2 months of maximum effort during which they were supposed to eat their diet exactly as specified, the study's participants were allowed to go their own way and select their own food. They were then followed for the next year.

The authors reported very modest average weight losses in all four diet groups, with the Atkins dieters having lost the least by the end of the year. They lost on average 4.6 lbs or 2% of their average starting weight. The dieters eating the very low fat Ornish diet did the best. They had an average loss at the end of the year of 7.3 lbs. The researchers concluded,

> Each diet significantly reduced the low-density lipoprotein/high-density lipoprotein (HDL) cholesterol ratio by approximately 10%, ... with no significant effects on blood pressure or glucose at 1 year. Amount of weight loss was associated with self-reported dietary adherence level but not with diet type.

In short, this study found that it didn't really matter which diet the dieters ate, as long as they stuck to a diet. However, almost half of those assigned to the more extreme diets—48% for Atkins and 50% for Ornish—dropped out of the study, compared to those who embarked on more moderate diets. Only 35% dropped out of the Zone group or Weight Watchers group.

The silver lining for Atkins dieters was that this large, prestigious study contradicted claims that eating the diet would worsen their cardiovascular health. This study showed that the Atkins diet had the same mildly positive effects on dieters' lipids as the other diets, though it did not live up to its claims to be superior for improving blood sugar or weight loss.

But what went unmentioned in any of the coverage of this study was a glaring fact you'll only discover if you read the full text of the study: The "Atkins" diet group in this study, who had been eating on average 238 grams of carbohydrates each day before they started the study, only ate a low carb diet for the *first month* of the study, and even then they never approached the carb intake levels prescribed by Dr. Atkins.

Over that first month the average carb intake of the "Atkins" group was 68 grams a day, with some participants reporting eating as many as 209 grams. By the second month, their average intake was 137 grams. By six months it was 190 grams, where it remained until the end of the year. Not only that, by the end of the year, about half of the Atkins dieters had gone off the diet completely.

The authors also point out that the weight loss achieved by those eating all the diets studied could be explained by the participants' reported calorie intake, which was taken to mean that there was no "metabolic advantage" to the Atkins diet, contrary to Dr. Atkins' claims. But since the "Atkins" dieters weren't eating an Atkins diet, this finding can be dismissed.

It is possible that a flaw in the methodology used to estimate the participants' food intake in this study may have overestimated how many carbs they were eating and produced an inaccurate total for their overall calorie intake, too. That's because the researchers collected information about what the participants ate by administering a standardized food questionnaire.

This multiple choice questionnaire is commonly used by nutritional researchers. It has been verified by studies that compare the estimates the questionnaire produces with the actual intake dieters come up with when they log their exact food intake.

The problem with the questionnaire is that it was developed and tested in groups of people eating high carb diets. As a result, its questions are phrased in a way that assumes that everyone filling in the survey is eating a substantial amount of carbohydrates. This makes it impossible to report a truly low carb intake.

I filled in just such a questionnaire, when I participated in a low carb diet study. The choices supplied in the form of multiple choice questions asked about my intake of bread, potatoes, and cereal in ways that made it impossible to answer that I had eaten only one or two servings of these foods during the course of the entire month. The smallest amounts I could select were always higher than those that a person would eat on a ketogenic low carb diet.

So it is hard to know exactly what this study proves, beyond the fact that people lost weight in accordance with the degree to which they stuck to their diets. If the questionnaire was at all accurate, it would suggest that many people who start out eating what they think is an Atkins-style, very low carb diet are not actually eating one, and that even the people who do manage to start off well end up eating a diet that can not be described as "low carb" after only a few months. Since other studies we'll look at next using different methodologies for tracking food intake came up with a similar finding, it is possible that few of the "Atkins" dieters in this study ate an Atkins diet for longer than a month or two.

A Major Problem with All Diet Research

Before we turn to our next study, it's also worth noting that there is a major flaw with this study and almost *all* diet studies that limits how much they can tell us about how effective any diet is for weight loss. The problem is that the only findings reported when the study is published are the average weight losses achieved by entire groups. These averages lose their meaning when you are talking about a group of dieters where a large number of people have stopped eating the diet being studied.

If you have a group where one person loses 50 lbs, one loses 15 lbs, one loses 10 and 7 go off their diet after a month and lose nothing, the average weight loss of these ten dieters group will be reported as 7.5 lbs which bears little relationship to the actual experiences of the dieters. So while this kind of reporting is useful for comparing diets, it doesn't help us know what kind of weight loss we might expect if we tried one of these diets. It also doesn't give us insight into the characteristics of the people who did manage to lose more weight than the average on a given diet.

The A to Z Study

A second, larger study that offered participants much more guidance as to how to do its diets was, "Comparison of the Atkins, Zone, Ornish, and LEARN Diets for Change in Weight and Related Risk Factors Among Overweight Premenopausal Women" published in the *Journal of the American Medical Association* in 2007, two years after the Tufts study. (Gardner, 2007)

This study, which was nicknamed the "A to Z" study—Atkins to Zone—was similar to the Tufts study, in that it tested the Atkins, Zone, and Ornish diets, to which it added another very low fat diet, the LEARN diet, which was similar to the Ornish diet but also required exercise.

This study followed 311 overweight or obese nondiabetic, premenopausal women who were put on one of the three diets for a year after being given a substantial amount of education about their assigned diet. The average starting weight of the Atkins dieters was 189 pounds. Their average age was 42. They received eight weekly one hour classes explaining how to do the diet and read the book, *Dr. Atkins' New Diet Revolution,* in conjunction with their weekly classes.

The people in the Atkins group in this study did a better job of sticking to their diets in the early months than had those in the Tufts study. A full 88% of the Atkins dieters completed the study, which was higher than the 77%, 76%, and 78% completion rates for the Zone, LEARN, and Ornish dieters.

At two months, the Atkins dieters' reported an average carbohydrate intake of 61 grams a day or 17.7% of all calories. By six months their average carbohydrate intake had risen to 113 grams a day or 29.5% of all their calories. Still, their caloric intake was, on average, about 350 calories a day less than it had been before they had started their diets, a decrease that should produce an average weight loss of three pounds a month.

By the end of the year, the average carbohydrate intake of the Atkins group had risen to 138 grams a day, or 34.5% of all their calories. Their calories had risen to where they were only 300 calories a day less than what they'd been eating before they'd started their diets.

The result of this Not-Quite-Atkins diet was an average loss of 10.34 pounds for the entire group, with individuals' losses mostly falling into the range between 7 and 14 lbs. This was considerably better than the weight loss achieved by the dieters on the other diets the A to Z study tested. For example, the Ornish dieters lost, on average, only 1.69 lbs. (Remember that these averages have to include the lack of weight loss experienced by people who gave up on the diet.)

The six months point, when the Atkins group was eating that average of 113 grams a day, was also the point where they achieved their maximum weight loss, which averaged almost 12 lbs. They then slowly started regaining over the next six months as their carbs continued to creep upwards. When this study analyzed the participants' cholesterol they reported:

> At all time points, the statistically significant findings for HDL-C and triglycerides concentrations favored the Atkins group. Changes in LDL-C concentrations at 2 months favored the LEARN and Ornish diets over the Atkins diet; however, these differences diminished and were no longer significant at 6 and 12 months.

In discussing the rise in LDL levels experienced by the Atkins dieters during the first two months of their diets the study explains,

> ... at 2 months, mean LDL-C concentrations increased by 2% and mean triglyceride concentrations decreased by 30% in the Atkins group. These findings are consistent with a beneficial increase in LDL particle size, although LDL particle size was not assessed in our study. In addition, we examined non–HDL-C concentrations as an alternate indicator of atherogenic lipoproteins—a variable not substantially influenced by changes in triglyceride concentrations—and observed no significant differences among groups at any time point.

This is very reassuring, because what it is saying is that though the Atkins dieters' LDL did rise at first—which is commonly reported by most dieters eating ketogenic diets, other factors changed in ways that suggested this rise was nothing to worry about. HDL and triglyceride improved in a way that suggested that the reason LDL was higher was because the LDL particles had become larger and healthier. It is well-known that it is the smaller, denser LDL particles that accumulate in our arteries and create the plaque that promotes heart disease. So increasing the size of LDL particles makes them less likely to clog arteries.

The Atkins dieters' blood pressure also decreased modestly, as did their fasting insulin. Though the researchers describe their subjects as healthy individuals with normal blood sugars, their average fasting blood sugar at the beginning of the study was at the *upper* end of the normal range, averaging 92 mg/dl. This range has been linked in epidemiological studies to a higher risk than normal of developing diabetes over time.[9]

However, the actual amount the Atkins dieters' average fasting blood sugar dropped over the study was not large, and not substantially different from the improvement the Zone dieters achieved, though it was better than that of the very low fat Ornish and LEARN dieters.

The Atkins group also started out with fasting insulin levels slightly higher than true normal, which dropped a very small amount after their year of dieting. But fasting insulin dropped by almost the identical amount in *all* groups of dieters except those eating the very high carbohydrate Ornish diet.

Unfortunately, these fasting glucose and fasting insulin measurements don't tell us what we'd really like to know: how did these dieters' blood sugars perform when they ate their meals? To learn that the subjects would have had to be given a meal test or a glucose tolerance test, but those tests weren't done, probably because of the expense. So this study tells us nothing about whether this diet made the kind of difference in blood sugar levels that would translate into less hunger and a lower risk of heart disease.

The Atkins dieters' blood pressure, which had been in the normal range to start with, also improved a little bit, as did that of the dieters in all the other groups. Though again the group eating the extremely low fat Ornish diet improved the least.

There is one other, very important thing this study teaches us: that you don't have to eat a ketogenic diet to lose weight and improve your health. The Atkins dieters eating a nonketogenic diet that provided on average 113 grams of carbohydrate a day ended up with improved health.

Their weight only started to rise from its 6 month low when they boosted their carbohydrate intake from an average of 113 grams to almost 140 grams a day. And even with that increase, these dieters maintained most of their weight loss. For most of them, that weight

---

[9] A study of 13,163 male soldiers followed over 12 years found that those with fasting blood sugars between 91 and 99 mg/dl at the beginning of the study were far more likely than others to develop diabetes. (Tirosh, 2005)

loss would have been fat not water and glycogen, because 113 grams a day is enough carbs to refill the glycogen stores of all but the most obese dieters.

This finding is important. As we'll see in Chapter 14, when we discuss the experience of people who have successfully maintained low carb weight losses for three years or more, many long-term low carbers report that they find it easiest to maintain their weight loss at a nonketogenic daily carbohydrate intake near 110 grams a day.

Some studies of people with diabetes using medications and anecdotal reports from people in the online diabetes community confirm that this intake level works well for many people with diabetes, too.

The Low Carb/Low Fat/Mediterranean Diet Study

A two-year long study which received a lot of attention in the medical press was titled, "Weight Loss with a Low-Carbohydrate, Mediterranean, or Low-Fat Diet." It was published in 2008 in the *New England Journal of Medicine.* (Shai, 2008)

This study too, found that the low carb diet produced superior weight loss and improvement in various measures of metabolic health. It did better than the Mediterranean diet in almost every respect— though the press reports about this study reported it almost exclusively as if it had pointed to the superior health benefits of the *Mediterranean* diet.

But I am not going to discuss it here because the tables of results included in this study shows that by six months into this study, the average carbohydrate intake of the entire "low carbohydrate" diet group was 40% of total calories. That would work out to 180 grams a day of carbohydrate for a male eating 1,800 calories or 150 grams for a woman eating 1,500.

This may mean that few people adhered to their low carb diets, but it is more likely to be a statistical issue caused by the fact that 29 people who didn't complete the full two years of the study had their data included in the tabulations. It is also possible that people who stopped eating their assigned diet may also have been included in the averages.

Whatever the case, though the low carb diet did very well in this study, it can tell us little about the impact of a low carb diet because of the way the data was presented.

The 2 Year Low Fat/Low Carb Comparison Study

A much better 2 year-long major comparison study, "Weight and Metabolic Outcomes After 2 Years on a Low-Carbohydrate Versus Low-

Fat Diet: A Randomized Trial" was published in 2010 in the journal, *Annals of Internal Medicine*. (Foster, 2010) The participants in this study were a mixed group. Roughly two thirds of them were female, with an average starting weight of 228 lbs. Their average age was roughly 50. None had diabetes and the authors did not report what their blood sugars had been at the beginning of the study. The low carb diet used in this study is described thus:

> During the first 12 weeks of treatment, participants were instructed to limit carbohydrate intake to 20 g/d in the form of low–glycemic index vegetables. After the first 12 weeks, participants gradually increased carbohydrate intake (5 g/d per week) by consuming more vegetables, a limited amount of fruits, and eventually small quantities of whole grains and dairy products, until a stable and desired weight was achieved. They followed guidelines described in Dr. Atkins' New Diet Revolution ... but were not provided with a copy of the book. Participants were instructed to focus on limiting carbohydrate intake and to eat foods rich in fat and protein until they were satisfied.

By the end of the first year, 26% of the original low carb dieters had stopped eating the diet. This was almost identical to the percentage of low fat dieters who had quit. By the end of two years, 42% of the low carb dieters had stopped, compared to 32% of the low fat dieters.

In this study, the researchers made no attempt to determine what the dieters had actually eaten. This is a major weakness and would make us wonder if, like the dieters in the 2003 study, these "low carb" dieters were not eating a low carb diet. However, the researchers did test for ketones in this study, and report that 63% of the low carb dieters tested positive for ketones at 3 months. At six months 28% tested positive for ketones.

The study does not report on the percentage of the low carb dieters who were showing ketones after that, but does remark that it was the same as for the low fat diet group. People burning body fat even when eating diets containing carbohydrate will spill some ketones, too, as will people who have been fasting since dinner without further snacking.

This would suggest that by one year all the dieters were eating well over the level where people start showing significant amounts of ketones in their urine, which is somewhere between 70 and 100 grams a day, though it is likely, given what we've seen in other studies, that they were eating a lot more.

Like the dieters in the A to Z study, the dieters in this study achieved their greatest weight loss at 6 months—an average of 25 lbs, which was roughly 11% of their starting weight. Over the next six months they gained back an average of 2 pounds, again mirroring the experience of the A to Z dieters.

But the A to Z study only lasted one year. This one went on for two, and at the end of that two years the Atkins dieters had gained back on average another 8 lbs compared to what they'd weighed at the end of one year of dieting. So their net loss over the two years averaged 16 lbs, or 7% of their average starting weight. Overall, they had lost and maintained, on average, only 2 lbs more than the low fat diet group did.

The conclusion we must draw once again from the limited information we are given in this study is that very few people can stick with a very low carb diet for two years. Maximum weight loss occurs by six months into the diet, after which, as people lose their motivation, they slowly regain the weight they've lost, though not all of it.

The reported values of the other health parameters in this study confirmed what the A to Z study had found: Cholesterol improved over the whole two years of the study, with LDL and VLDL dropping and HDL rising. During the very early months when most of the low carb dieters were eating a ketogenic low carb diet, as shown by their ketone status, their triglycerides dropped the most, after which they began to rise, but at the end of the study, they were still better than they'd been before their diets began. Blood pressure also improved slightly, and was best early on, rising as carbohydrate intake did, though it, too, was still better at the end of the study than it had been before the study began.

Because nutritionists have been warning for years that a diet high in protein will damage bone, this study also measured the participants' bone density and found no sign of any significant changes in bone density after two years.

The Australian Calorie-Controlled Study

None of these large well-publicized studies tells us much about what happens when people eat a ketogenic diet for more than a month or two, since, by design, they all raised the participants' carbohydrate intake level to a level high enough to refill their glycogen stores after a very brief introductory period where they ate a ketogenic diet.

But a study that was ignored by the health media fills that gap. It not only studied a long-term ketogenic diet, it also addressed the question of whether there is, as has been claimed by Dr. Atkins and others, a "metabolic advantage" to eating a ketogenic low carb as opposed to a low fat or low calorie diet.

This study, "Long-term effects of a very-low-carbohydrate weight loss diet compared with an isocaloric low-fat diet after 12 mo," was conducted in Australia. It ensured that its 188 subjects were eating the diet the researchers intended to study by giving them classes, consultations with nutritionists, food plans, coaching, training in how to estimate the nutritional content of what they were eating, opportunities to support each other, and most importantly, free food.

Each group was given food that fit the parameters of their assigned diet, enough to provide to one third of their daily nutritional needs for the first two months of the study. They also received a cash supplement each month to help with their food expenses. (Brinkworth, 2009)

Not surprisingly, given this level of support, the participants in this study who stuck with their diets did far better than did the subjects in any of the other diet studies we looked at. Instead of stopping after five or six months, their weight loss continued throughout the study's entire year.

But despite, or perhaps even *because* of the support they got, which enabled them to adhere to their diets, but which also must have put more pressure on them to do so, 42% of the low carb dieters in this Australian study dropped out as did 41% of the low fat dieters. The dieters who dropped out of both arms of the study tended to be slightly heavier than those who persisted. This reinforces the fact that even under ideal conditions, with a lot more support than most people will ever get, long-term dieting on any diet is tough.

The low carb diet prescribed here limited not only the dieter's carbs but also their calories, since one goal of the study was to compare how the low carb dieters fared when compared to a group of low fat dieters eating the exact same number of calories each day. Doing this would, it was hoped, determine whether the metabolic improvements the low carb diet had produced in other trials were actually due to its nutrient makeup or if they occurred because dieters ended up eating a lot less calories due to the low carb diet's ability to reduce hunger.

The daily calorie intake target for women was set at 1,433 calories and for men at 1,672. The low carb diet group was to get 4% of its total energy from carbohydrate, 35% from protein, and 61% from total fat (20% saturated fat) with the objective of restricting carbohydrate intake to less than 20 grams per day for the first 8 weeks and to less than 40 grams a day for the remainder of the study.

The dieters' urinary ketones were tested periodically to validate that they were, in fact, eating a ketogenic diet. Though their ketone levels declined throughout the study, especially after the dieters raised their carbohydrate intake to the 40 gram a day level, some level of ketones was detected in all the low carb dieters who remained in the study throughout the year.

It is worth noting that the low *fat* dieters in this study also showed ketones—a sign that they, too, were burning fat—but their ketone levels were lower than those the low carb dieters. This would be expected since the low fat dieters were burning much less *dietary* fat.

The low carb group was two thirds female and averaged 51.5 years of age. It lost more weight, on average, than the low fat group throughout the study. Both groups dropped a lot of weight during the first 8 weeks. The low carb group lost an average of approximately 17 lbs, which was almost 3 lbs more than the low fat group, though this difference could easily be attributed to their lost glycogen.

Weight loss slowed down for both groups after that initial burst of weight loss. At 6 months, the low carb group had lost, on average, another 13 pounds, while the low fat group had lost, on average, another 10. And though weight loss continued after that first 6 months, which is where this study differs from all the others we examined, the actual average weight loss that took place in both the low carb and low fat group over that second 6 month period was very small compared to their weight loss during the first 6 months —less than 3 lbs, which works out to half a pound a month for both groups.

At the end of the year-long study, those in the low carb group who had stayed on plan for the whole year had achieved an average weight loss of 31.9 lbs, with most individual weight loss amounts falling in a range between 28.2 and 35.6 lbs. Since the average starting weight of this group was 207 lbs, this average loss represents a loss of 15% of their average starting weight.

On average, too, by the end of the study the low carb group had lost approximately ten more pounds than did the low fat group, though both groups had been eating the same number of calories daily. You can see a graph displaying this weight loss data at:

http://www.ajcn.org/content/90/1/23/F3.expansion.html

It is difficult to determine if this difference in weight loss could be attributed to glycogen loss. The researchers state that the changes in body composition between the two groups were not significantly different, but the method they used to estimate body composition, dual-energy X-ray absorptiometry (DEXA) is one that may give inaccurate results in glycogen-depleted low carb dieters. (Manninen, 2006)

In this study, blood pressure, fasting glucose, fasting insulin, and a computed measure of insulin resistance all improved over time in *both* groups with no discernable differences due to either the choice of diet or the dieters' sex.

Most significantly, variations in these variables corresponded to the *amount of weight loss*, not which diet the dieters had eaten. C-reactive protein (CRP), a measure of inflammation, also decreased equally in both diet groups, with no variation attributable to the differences in the diets or the dieters' gender.

Both groups in this study started the diet with an average fasting blood sugar that would put them in the prediabetic range (103 mg/dl for the low carb group, and 101 mg/dl for the low fat group.) At the end of the study the average fasting glucose in each group had dropped by the same small amount to a level that, while technically normal, was at the very top of the normal range. Both groups' average fasting insulin was elevated at the beginning of the study, too, and dropped by almost the same amount, though the low fat group had started out with an average fasting insulin that was significantly higher than that of the low carb group. This suggests strongly that either weight loss or food restriction, rather than diet composition, is what lowers fasting insulin.

As was the case in the previous studies we examined, the low carb diet in this study led to greater increases in total cholesterol, LDL cholesterol, and HDL cholesterol and to a bigger reduction in triglycerides than did the low fat diet. As in the A to Z study, the authors said, "This suggests that the increase in LDL cholesterol with an LC diet may be due to an increase in LDL cholesterol particle size as well as particle number." These lipid changes did *not* vary with either how many calories the individual low carb dieters consumed or how much weight they had lost.

In the end, the researchers concluded that it was impossible to determine whether the differences in weight loss between the low carb and low fat dieters could be attributed to the different composition of the diets since, because of the high number of drop outs, the number of participants who completed the study wasn't large enough to eliminate the possibility that the weight loss gap might have been due to chance. With only 33 low carb dieters completing the study, the average weight loss of the group could have been skewed by the random inclusion of a few outliers.

It is also likely, though the authors do not discuss this possibility, that at least some of that excess 10 pound weight loss achieved by dieters in the low carb diet group was partly due to glycogen depletion, since the dieters in this study stuck to their ketogenic diets, unlike those in the other studies we looked at.

Another Problem with All Diet Research

The weight loss statistics you find in these and all other diet studies may be misleading, not only because they are given as averages, but because in order to be considered scientifically valid, researchers must test these diets in groups of *randomly chosen* people who have in common only that they hope to lose weight.

This means in each diet study group there are people for whom the diet they must eat is completely wrong. They may hate the food. The dietary requirements may be difficult to integrate into their work or social life. The diet may have some subtle effect on their physiology that makes them feel wretched. And of course, many placed on a very low carb diet will, in fact, have completely normal blood sugars, so they won't experience the hunger-quieting effect of the low carb diet that makes it so attractive to people whose abnormal blood sugars make them get hungry on high carb diets.

So it's possible that when people are free to select their own diets, the people who choose a low carb diet will be those who find the food appealing and feel better on it. They would be more likely to stick with their diets than the dieters in these study groups, and might do better, both in terms of how much weight they lose and in how well their blood sugar improves.

Points to Remember from This Chapter:

1. Figure 6 on Page 60 summarizes the typical weight loss curves reported in these studies.

Average weight loss on low carb diets, no matter how motivated, educated, or supported the dieters might be, starts off fast, slows dramatically by six months, and proceeds at a crawl thereafter, if it doesn't entirely stop.

2. Keeping carbohydrates under 115 grams a day should prevent weight regain, but even eating at a lower carbohydrate intake does not ensure the kind of speedy ongoing weight loss most dieters hope to achieve in return for stringently controlling their eating.

3. Nonketogenic low carb diets also produce weight loss and achieve the health benefits claimed for the ketogenic diet, especially those that limit carbohydrate intakes to a level near 110 grams a day.

4. Low carb diets do appear to improve cholesterol profiles better than other diets at least over the short-term.

5. Though the weight losses on a strict ketogenic diet will be better than those on a laxer one, strict diets may be tougher to stick to.

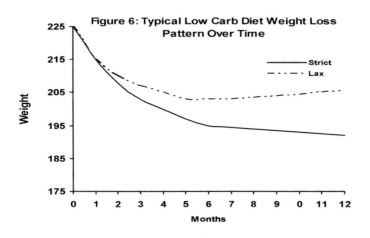

6. No matter how well they stick to a strict ketogenic diet, most people will have to settle for a modest weight loss of no more than 15% of their starting weight. Most of that weight loss will occur in the first few months of the diet, after which it will slow dramatically. When weight loss slows, dieters are more prone to become lax about their diets.

Chapter 4

Filling in the Details

The large, long-term studies we just looked at focused mainly on establishing the safety and effectiveness of the low carb diet. To learn more about the specifics we have to turn to smaller, often shorter, studies that flesh out our understanding of how the diet affects the people who eat it.

Individual Responses to a Ketogenic Diet and the Diet's Side Effects

A small, relatively short study of the Atkins diet was published in 2004 by a team at Duke University that included Dr. Eric Westman, who later went on to become one of the authors of the revised version of the officially sanctioned Atkins diet book, *The New Atkins for a New You*. This study is useful because it gives insight into how individuals do on the diet, rather than just presenting a group's average performance. (Yancy, 2004)

A chart included with this study, which you can view at:

http://www.annals.org/content/140/10/769/F3.expansion.html

shows that weight loss started to slow for many of the Atkins dieters as early as the 12th week after they had begun their diets. It also demonstrates that the heavier dieters in the study, whose weight was close to 300 lbs at the study's start, experienced much larger weight losses than did those whose starting weights were under 200.

This is the kind of finding that is impossible to extract from the studies that present only averages. The Duke group is to be commended for providing this rare example of actual patient data.

The other thing this Duke study does is give a list of the side effects the low carb dieters encountered in the course of their ketogenic diets. They included, constipation (present in 68% of the dieters), headache (60%), bad breath (38%), muscle cramps (35%), diarrhea (23%), general weakness (25%), and rash (13%)

We'll discuss all these side effects and the best way to remedy them in Chapter 11.

How Low Carb Affects Mood and Brain Function

Another informative study was published by the same Australian group whose elegant year-long study we discussed in the previous chapter. It attempted to find out if the ketogenic diet has a negative impact on brain function. This is an important question, because nutritionists have been telling patients for years that unless the brain gets over 100 grams of glucose a day it won't function properly. (Brinkworth, 2009)

As you'll recall, many of the dieters in that Australian study ate a ketogenic low carb diet for the entire year the study lasted and achieved a continuing weight loss throughout that year, unlike participants in the other diet studies we looked at.

The researchers observed that during the first few months of their diet, the people eating the ketogenic diet experienced improved brain function, and their average scores for anxiety, depression, and anger decreased, when tested by various standardized tests. But over the course of the year, most of the measures used to gauge their mood returned to what they had been at the start of the study.

Only one measure, that of anger, ended up slightly higher in the low carb diet group than it had been at the start of the study. In contrast, the low fat dieters' average measures of mood improved early on and stayed more positive throughout the year.

The authors speculate that this difference in the two groups might have been due in part to the fact that the dieters had been randomly assigned to the different diets rather than being allowed to choose the diet that best fit their food preferences. They also comment that the low carbohydrate diet is more difficult to adhere to in a society where carbohydrates play such a large part in social interaction. As they put it in their published paper,

> Therefore, the LC diet being so far removed from normal dietary habits may have created a significant challenge for participants, leading to the possibility of food preoccupation, social eating impairment, and dysphoria. Although, in the short term, participants may have been able to meet the challenges presented by this dietary pattern, over the longer term, it may have increased participant isolation, leading to the negative impact on mood state that may provide a possible explanation for the effects that were observed.

This is an astute observation and should not be dismissed. The high level of attrition in *all* low carb diet studies shows that many people *do* find it very hard to adhere to the diet long-term. But the authors also point out that despite the differences between the two diet groups, the low carb dieters' test results on the mood tests were all still well within normal limits.

When the researchers turned to the question of whether putting the brain into a ketogenic state decreased thinking ability, they found that "... after 8 weeks, obese participants on an LC diet had less improvement in speed of processing (inspection time task) but similar improvements in working memory compared with obese participants on a conventional low fat diet."

This study got some play in the media since it appeared to confirm the prejudices of stubborn anti-fat crusaders who had been hitherto hard-pressed to find any negatives in the research studying low carb diets. But the actual phrasing makes it clear that what the researchers are saying here is that the low carb dieters' average processing speed didn't *improve*. They did *not* report that it decreased.

And any deficit in the speed of mental processing of low carb dieters compared to that of the people eating a low fat diet disappeared as the year progressed. The researchers concluded, "...any decrements in cognitive performance following introduction to an LC diet are transient and short-lived." Not only that, but "the improvement in working memory, as assessed by DSB [the "digit span backward" test], that occurred after 8 weeks was sustained over 12 months in both diet groups."

To sum up their findings, one year of eating a ketogenic diet made dieters a bit testier, though it did not otherwise affect their mood. It slightly improved their cognitive performance, though the people eating a low fat diet experienced the same results.

Low Carb Diets and Insulin Levels in Insulin Resistant Dieters

A claim, which has been repeated so often in low carb diet books that it is generally believed to be true, is that low carb diets are superior to other diets because of the way they lower insulin and reverse insulin resistance. However, a well-conducted 24 week study that put three groups of middle-aged, obese, insulin resistant women on either an Atkins-style low carb diet, the Zone diet (called a High Protein diet in the study), or a high fiber/high carbohydrate diet provides us with some data with which to check this claim.

The study was titled, "Comparison of high-fat and high-protein diets with a high-carbohydrate diet in insulin-resistant obese women." In this study the participants' dietary intake was estimated by giving them food scales and having them report their daily input periodically. It lasted 24 weeks or roughly 6 months. (McAuley, 2005)

At 8 weeks the low carb dieters' average daily carbohydrate intake was 41 grams. At 16 and 24 weeks they reported eating an average intake of 106 and 107 grams a day. When it was measured at 8 weeks, their average weight had declined. It then stayed very stable for the rest of the study. This was true for participants on all three diets. The low carb dieters lost a few more pounds on average than the other dieters, but they also ended up eating about 40 calories a day less than did the high carb dieters, which would explain that difference.

Since the low carb dieters in this study were eating a ketogenic low carb diet for the first eight weeks of the study and a nonketogenic low carb diet for the rest of it, the changes in their insulin levels and fasting blood sugars should tell us something about the effects of both kinds of diet on insulin resistance, as indeed they do.

Figure 7 shows charts based on data presented in tables published with this study. As you can see at the start of the study all three groups had similar average fasting blood sugars, though the low carb and Zone dieters were on average slightly higher at approximately 92 mg/dl compared to the 90 mg/dl of the low fat dieters.

At the start of the study, the average fasting insulin of the Atkins group was also very similar to that of the group that went on to eat the high carb/low fat diet. But unlike those in other studies, the researchers in this study also administered the 2-hour oral glucose tolerance test, which gives us a better idea of whether the diet really improved blood sugar control than do fasting insulin and fasting glucose.

Before the study began, the average 2-hour glucose tolerance test results of the Atkins diet group was higher, at 106 mg/dl, than that of the other two diet groups, though still well within the normal range. Nevertheless, this small difference might suggest that, overall, the Atkins dieters were slightly more insulin resistant than the other two groups.

Eight weeks into the diet the fasting blood sugars of the Atkins dieters had dropped to a more normal 86 mg/dl. But so did the fasting blood sugars of the dieters eating a *high carb*, high fiber diet—even though they did not end up eating as much fiber as they had been told to eat. Both groups saw their fasting glucose remain at this new, improved level for the rest of the study, though the fasting blood sugar of the low fat dieters continued to decrease slightly, while that of the low carb dieters stayed constant. The Zone dieters' fasting blood sugars dropped only a very small amount.

Fasting Blood Sugar

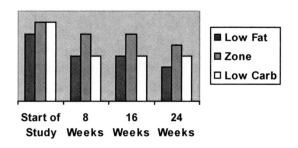

2-Hr Blood Sugar

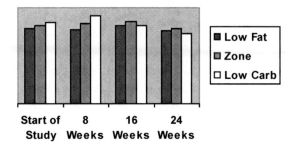

Fasting Insulin

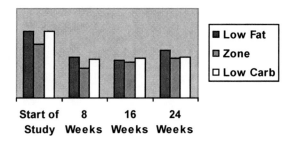

Figure 7. Changes in Blood Sugar and Insulin

At this same 8 week point, when the low carb dieters were mostly eating a ketogenic diet, their average 2 hour glucose tolerance test result rose to 115 mg/dl, which was 9 mg/dl *higher* than their average test result before they started the diet.

This is not a surprise. Dieters who are eating a very low carb diet need to "carb up" for three days before taking a glucose tolerance test or their readings will be artificially high. This happens because they have downregulated some of the hormones needed to digest complex carbohydrates and burn glucose, since their bodies have been almost exclusively burning fats.

However, at 16 and 24 weeks when the low carb dieters had raised their carbohydrate intake so that they were no longer eating a ketogenic diet, their 2-hour glucose tolerance test result dropped *below* its starting value and it continued to drop for the rest of the study.

At 24 weeks their 2-hour glucose tolerance test result was, on average, a solid 92 mg/dl, which was a decrease of 14 mg/dl from their starting value. The dieters on the other diets saw smaller decreases in their average 2 h GTT results — about 4 mg/dl by the end of the study. But since they had started out with lower readings, the differences between their readings and those of the Atkins dieters were small. The average fasting insulin of the Atkins dieters dropped the most at the 8 week point, but what is interesting is that *the average fasting insulin of the high carb dieters dropped, too* and was very similar to that of the Atkins dieters.

At 16 weeks, after the Atkins dieters had raised their carbs out of the ketogenic range, their fasting insulin started to rise, while that of the high carb dieters continued to drop, even though they were eating on average 171 grams of carbohydrate a day, compared to the 106 eaten by the low carb dieters. At the end of the study, the average fasting insulin of the high carb group had risen slightly more than that of the low carb dieters, though the low carb dieters' fasting insulin had also risen very slightly.

Though there were differences between how all three diet groups did on average, these differences were small, and all three diet groups ended up with very similar changes in all three measures of blood sugar health. This suggests that the argument that the low carb diet is the *only* diet that lowers insulin levels may be wrong, since the insulin levels of both high and low carb dieters in this study improved in ways that were very similar. But it does appear that a moderately low carb

diet improves how blood sugars perform after meals in people with normal or only very slightly abnormal blood sugars.

The Rest of the Story . . . A Cautionary Tale

Read on its own, this study would suggest that, while it might not make any major or permanent change in insulin levels or insulin resistance, the low carb diet is as effective for improving blood sugar control as any other diet that causes weight loss. However, the same team published a *follow-up* study the next year, which tells a more cautionary tale. This study was given the title, "Long-term effects of popular dietary approaches on weight loss and features of insulin resistance." (McAuley, 2006)

When the six months of the original study were over, the dieters were instructed to stay on their diets. Then they were called back six months later for another examination. By this time all the dieters on all the plans had gone off their diets. The erstwhile Akins dieters now reported eating, on average, 147 grams of carbohydrate a day which was only 13 grams a day less than what the high carbohydrate diet group was eating.

Unfortunately for the Atkins dieters, though they had raised their carbohydrate intake out of the range most people would consider low carb, they had *not* lowered their fat intake from the very high level that is appropriate *only* when eating a ketogenic diet. So their fat intake—87 grams a day—was much higher than that of either of the other groups. Because of their higher fat intake, the Atkins dieters' daily calorie intake was now 200 calories a day higher than that of the Zone dieters' and 300 higher than that of the low fat dieters.

Not surprisingly, over the six months since they'd ended their diets, the erstwhile Atkins dieters had regained *more fat mass and more waist circumference* than had the Zone dieters. Even though the Atkins dieters had originally lost more weight than the low fat dieters, a year after the start of their diets they ending up weighing very close to what the low fat dieters weighed. However, because they were gaining weight at a much faster rate than the low fat dieters, due to eating that extra 300 calories a day, it was very likely that in another six months the erstwhile Atkins dieters would weigh considerably more than the low fat dieters, since the low fat dieters were regaining at a much slower rate.

The LDL cholesterol of the erstwhile Atkins dieters had remained higher than the LDL the other groups, too, once they had gone off their diets, but their triglycerides had risen in a way that suggested that their LDL level was no longer high because it was made up of the large, fluffy molecules considered healthy.

And though their average fasting insulin level was still better than it had been when they'd started their diets, as were the fasting insulin levels of all three groups of dieters, the erstwhile Atkins dieters' average 2 hour reading on the glucose tolerance test had gone back up almost to its starting level, which suggests that their diets had made no meaningful change to either their insulin resistance or their blood sugar control.

In this study, the dieters who fared the best when they went *off* their diets were the Zone dieters who had been eating a diet that was 40% carbs, 30% protein, and 30% fat during the period when they had been sticking to their diets. They ended up with the best weight loss at the end of the year, the best maintenance of their weight loss after they relaxed their diets, the most improved blood sugars, and the best lipids.

The Lesson to Be Learned

This study points out the single biggest danger of the ketogenic diet: It trains people to eat high levels of fat that are only healthful when they are keeping their carbohydrate intake very low. Because so few people stick to any diet for more than a few months, the low carb diet *may* be dangerous—not when people are eating it, but when they *abandon* it and take away from their dieting experience only the message that eating a lot of fat is healthy.

If you are going to succeed, long-term, on a low carb diet of any type, you must bear in mind that as you raise your carbs, you must cut back on fat. Once your carb intake goes over 150 grams of carbohydrate you'd be better off eating a diet closer to that of the Zone dieters, where 40% of calories come from carbs and only 30% from fat. For a person eating 2,000 calories a day, that would be only 67 grams of fat.

Otherwise, if you keep eating a lot of fat with that 150+ grams of carbs each day, you will justify the warnings of the fat-phobes who warn that a low carb diet will give you heart disease. It won't while you are eating it. But if your low carb/high fat diet becomes a high carb/high fat diet you *are* asking for serious trouble.

Low Carb Diets and Type 2 Diabetes

Though there are many people online who control their blood sugar using carb restriction, there is not much good data about the effects of eating a very low carb diet on people with Type 2 diabetes. Most of the studies we have that focus solely on people with diabetes are very short—only a few weeks long—or very small—following less than 20 and sometimes less than 10 subjects. These numbers are so low that the presence of a few outliers could greatly influence the result.

The few longer-term studies that were done using people with diabetes, like all the other studies we just discussed, are of limited value because they report their results only as averages and include in those averages data from those in the study population who weren't actually eating the diet.

Even so, it is possible to extract a few useful points from some of these studies. One was conducted by Dr. Westman and his Atkins-funded team at Duke. It was titled, "The effect of a low-carbohydrate, ketogenic diet versus a low-glycemic index diet on glycemic control in Type 2 diabetes mellitus." (Westman, 2008)

In this study the participants appear to have been eating a truly ketogenic diet through the 24 weeks the brief study lasted. It found that "there was no correlation between change in hemoglobin A1C and change in weight." If you'll recall, the A1C is a blood test that doctors believe reflects your average blood sugar over the previous three months.[10]

This finding, that the changes in the A1C did not correlate with changes in its subjects' weight, is very important, because doctors continue to tell people with diabetes that weight loss will improve their blood sugars. Some even claim that weight loss will reverse diabetes. But this study makes it clear that this is not true, which confirms what I've heard reported by almost all the people with diabetes I've polled.

Most have found that weight loss has little effect on their blood sugar control. Cutting down on carbs makes an immediate improvement in their blood sugars long before weight loss occurs—and long after it stops. But even significant weight losses rarely change the ability of most people with diabetes to control their blood sugars. And most find that no matter how much weight they lose, they still can't eat any more carbohydrate if they want to maintain normal blood sugars.

---

[10] The A1C test doesn't actually measure your blood sugar; instead it measures how much glucose is permanently bonded to the hemoglobin in your red blood cells. Since red blood cells usually live 3 months, in theory, this gives an indication of how much glucose those blood cells have been exposed to.

The A1C is a cheap way to gauge how well a person is controlling their blood sugar, though it is much less accurate than monitoring those same blood sugars with a meter. Genetic variations affecting how many red blood cells a person has and how those cells live can produce A1C results that don't match actual blood sugar readings collected over time by a Continuous Glucose Monitor.

Figure 8 below reproduces a chart published with the study that documents this clearly.

A 1% drop in A1C reflects a drop in average blood sugar of 28 mg/dl, which is quite large. As you can see, only 2 people eating the ketogenic diet (LCKD) saw their A1C go up, as compared to 11 people eating the high carb, "low glycemic" diet (LGID). We will return to the subject of the Glycemic Index in Chapter 6.

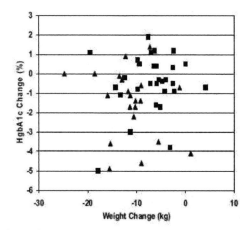

Graph reproduced from Westman, E C et al.:The effect of a low-carbohydrate, ketogenic diet versus a low-glycemic index diet on glycemic control in type 2 diabetes mellitus. *Nutrition & Metabolism* 2008, 5:36 doi:10.1186/1743-7075-5-36

Figure 8

Relationship between change in hemoglobin A1c and change in weight. This figure plots the change in hemoglobin A1c vs. the change in weight from baseline to week 24 for each individual (r = 0.09425, p = 0.5150). The LCKD group is shown as triangles; the LGID group is shown as squares.

However, there are some problems with this study. It is much easier to achieve a large improvement in A1C when you start out with a very high A1C. So the amount by which an individual's A1C has dropped is not a useful measure unless it is presented with information about what the individual's starting A1Cs had been, which was not included here.

But a far bigger problem with this study is that even though some subjects saw a dramatic drop in their A1C, most did not, and this was a group of people who started the study with an average A1C high enough to cause all the major diabetic complications.

After almost six months of eating their ketogenic diets, the average drop in the subjects' A1C was not enough to bring their blood sugars to a truly normal and safe blood sugar level. Many of them might have ended up much healthier if they had not depended so heavily on diet to lower their severely diabetic blood sugars. Had they worked with a skilled endocrinologist to come up with a properly designed insulin regimen that matched their insulin doses to the carbohydrate content of each meal, they would have been more likely to achieve truly normal blood sugars.[11]

But the biggest problem with this study is that, just as was the case in all the other studies we have looked at, almost half the participants stopped eating the diet before the 24 weeks were out. When dieters who diet for weight loss go off their diets, the worst that happens is that they end up having to buy bigger pants. But people with diabetes who can't stick to their diets can end up facing blindness, amputation, kidney failure, and heart attacks. So it's essential they adopt a diet that they can stick to for decades without needing superhuman amounts of willpower.

This stringent ketogenic diet failed too many people for it to be a good fit for most people with Type 2 diabetes, especially since the people in this study received more support than your average person with diabetes will receive.

The experience of the online diabetes community suggests that while some people do very well on a ketogenic low carb diet and stick to it for years, they can do this because they enjoy eating that way and don't have to struggle to stick to their diets. Those who do struggle are better off when they combine a diet slightly higher in carbohydrates— one that comes in nearer to 110 grams a day, which is much easier to eat in real world situations—with carefully chosen, safely dosed, diabetic medications.

This study was also brief, as it lasted only five and a half months. As we saw in the previous chapters, the first six months of any low carb diet is a honeymoon period whose gains are rarely maintained as the diet continues. That makes you wonder how the people with diabetes in this study would have done after more time had passed.

---

[11] Though some of the subjects in the study were using insulin, their poor results, coupled with what I've heard from many people with Type 2 diabetes, makes me suspect that the insulin regimens their family doctors prescribed were generic, "one size fits all" regimens that don't dose insulin to match carbohydrate intake, which is what a well-constructed insulin regimen should do. Many people with type 2 diabetes are only given long acting insulins like Lantus that affect only their fasting blood sugar. Those kinds of insulin don't do a good job of lowering blood sugars after meals. To do that, you need to use a fast-acting insulin. The best guide to how to use insulin with a low carb diet is the book, *Dr. Bernstein's Diabetes Solution*, by Dr. Richard K. Bernstein.

As it turns out, we have another study that gives us a better idea of what happens to people with diabetes who eat a carbohydrate-restricted diet over a longer period of time. This study was titled, "Effects of a Low-intensity Intervention That Prescribed a Low-carbohydrate vs. a Low-fat Diet in Obese, Diabetic Participants." (Iqbal, 2007) This trial lasted two years and followed a group of low carb dieters with poorly controlled diabetes who were advised to eat a diet of less than 30 grams a day of carbohydrate.

To help these dieters understand how much carbohydrate was in the foods they usually ate, they were counseled and provided with CalorieKing nutritional software, which does a very good job of calculating and tracking the carbs, calories, and other nutrients found in a wide selection of foods. The subjects were not told to restrict fat or calories, though they were counseled to eat more unsaturated fats.

Even more dieters dropped out of the low carb arm of this study over its two years than left the Duke diabetes study—60%, and that was considerably more than 46% who dropped out of the study's other arm, in which participants were advised to lower their calories by 500 a day and keep their fat intake to only 7% of all calories.

Dietary intake w0as estimated by asking the participants to report the specifics of their meals, snacks, and all other food intake over the previous 24 hours, but this was only done three times during the entire study. The average weight loss of the low carb dieters with diabetes peaked at 6 months, as was the case in the other studies we saw. Then their weight started creeping up so that at the end of the study the average weight loss of the low carb dieters was only 3.3 lbs.

More importantly, the long-term impact of the diet on these diabetic people's blood sugar echoed the weight loss. Their average A1C declined at 6 months but by a year it was back to almost where it had been when the study began. It was at that same level a year later. The low fat group achieved a slightly better improvement in both their average A1Cs and fasting glucose, but they still ended up with an average A1C high enough to almost guarantee they would develop some serious diabetic complications.

By now you can probably guess why the results of this study were so disappointing. Just like most of the low carb dieters in the other studies we examined, these "low carb" dieters with diabetes appear to have eaten a low carb diet for only the first few months of the study — the period during which they achieved that weight loss typical of low carb diets.

By the time they'd been eating their diets for 6 months their carbohydrate intake had risen to where it was only 4.7% less than what they'd been eating before they started their diets. Carbohydrates made up a full 35% of their daily intake. That would be 175 grams of carbohydrate a day for someone eating 2,000 calories a day. But these obese people with diabetes had *not* been told to lower their calories, so many of them would have been eating far more calories and carbs than that.

In contrast to most low carb dieters, these dieters did *not* raise their fat intake significantly, probably because people with diabetes are continually told that eating fat will kill them. Nor were they eating more protein.

Their carbohydrate intake only continued to deteriorate as the study progressed. At the end of the year they were eating almost as much carbohydrate as they had been at the study's start. And by the end of *two* years they were eating almost 8% *more* carbohydrate than they had been eating *before* they started what was supposed to be a very low carb diet.

Even more oddly, at the end of the study the "low carb" diet group had cut their *fat* intake more than the "low fat" diet group.

Taken together these findings reinforce the message I've been sharing with the diabetes community online for the past seven years. Cutting carbs is one of *many* tools available to people with diabetes, not the only one. Low carb diets work very well for a subset of people who enjoy eating the foods they provide and can adapt them to their lifestyles. Others will find they do better with a slightly higher carb intake, along with carefully chosen, safe and tested diabetes drugs. Many do best with a combination of injecting insulin and eating a diet that lowers carbs modestly. I discuss all these tools extensively in my book, *Blood Sugar 101* and on the web site of the same name, where you can find guidance on what to do if diet alone isn't enough to give you normal blood sugars.

If you have diabetes, keep in mind that hundreds, if not thousands, of people with diabetes who participate in online discussion groups *do* achieve excellent control over many years and avoid developing complications by using some combination of a diet that cuts back carbohydrates moderately—not extremely, along with some combination of safe oral drugs, insulin, and, when possible, exercise. Find the combination that works for you and you will, too.

Low Carb Diets and Fatty Liver Disease

You may have read that eating a ketogenic low carb diet will reverse nonalcoholic fatty liver disease (NAFLD). This is a condition, quite common among heavy people, that is diagnosed when blood tests come back showing higher than normal levels of liver enzymes.

When you have NAFLD, the cells in your liver have become clogged with triglycerides, the fat molecules that the liver makes out of excess glucose and fructose. The title of a recent study, "Intrahepatic fat, not visceral fat, is linked with metabolic complications of obesity" reflects the growing belief among scientists that it is this intracellular liver fat that causes insulin resistance and the other negative effects that were ascribed to visceral fat in the past. (Fabbrini, 2009)

Diets high in fructose contribute heavily to the formation of this intracellular liver fat, not just in people with blood sugar problems, but in normal people. (Lê, 2009) Most of the fructose we consume comes not from fruit, as many people wrongly believe, but from sugar and corn syrup.

There is some research that suggests that people eating a ketogenic low carb diet burn off more of this liver fat than do people eating low calorie diets that are not ketogenic. (Browning, 2008)

One finding that seems to back this up is that people diagnosed with NAFLD who are eating low carb diets will often see their liver enzymes drop back into the normal range. However, it turns out that the blood level of these liver enzymes is a poor indicator of how much actual fat you have stored in your liver. It is possible to lower the levels of these enzymes in your blood without actually decreasing your store of liver fat or the amount of scarring in your liver. (Chan, 2007)

The only accurate way of gauging how much liver fat you are carrying is to biopsy your liver—to open it up, take out a slice, and see what it looks like under the microscope. Needless to say, this isn't something your doctor is going to suggest anytime soon. However, when dieters are scheduled for other abdominal surgeries, alert researchers do take a snip out of their livers and examine them to see what effect various interventions may have made on their fatty livers.

One such biopsy study found that taking the insulin-sensitizing drug metformin, though it lowered the levels of liver enzymes, did not reduce the amount of liver fat. (Haukeland, 2009)

Another small study, run by a team from Dr. Westman's clinic at Duke, did liver biopsies on five people, four of whom had been eating a ketogenic diet for six months. It found that the dieters who had lost a lot of weight on their ketogenic diets did experience decreases in their liver fat as well as reductions in liver inflammation and fibrosis [scarring]. (Tendler, 2007)

However, because there was no control group in this study who had lost a similar amount of weight on a nonketogenic diet, it is impossible to know if the improvement in the subjects' livers came from eating a ketogenic diet or if it was caused by the large weight loss the subjects had experienced.

There is another recent liver biopsy study of dieters eating a low *fat* diet that followed a much larger group of dieters. It found that the degree of improvement in its subjects' NAFLD correlated directly with how much weight they had lost. Dieters who had lost 9% or more of their starting weight showed significant improvements in all the factors associated with fatty liver disease. (Harrison, 2009)

Both these studies found improvements in insulin resistance in all the subjects who had lost more than 5% of their starting weight. However, these studies, like so many others, determined insulin resistance using the HOMA formula, rather than by measuring the dieters' actual response to insulin.[12] So all they really tell us is that fasting insulin dropped, which will happen when you eat less food of *any* type. It can't tell us whether their insulin had become more efficient at disposing of the carbohydrate that comes in at meal-time.

If you have been diagnosed with NAFLD and are concerned about it, the good news is that a recent, huge, long-lasting epidemiological study has found that, contrary to what doctors have long told patients, a diagnosis of NAFLD appears to makes no difference in how long you'll live.

The researchers in this study analyzed data from more than 11,000 Americans between the ages of 20 to 74 who were followed for up to 18 years as part of the Third National Health and Nutrition Examination Survey (NHANES). They found no evidence of any increased risk of death among the 20% of participants who had been diagnosed with NAFLD. (Lazo, 2011) So while you will want to reduce your liver fat, in the hope that this might decrease your insulin resistance, it's good to know it does not pose the same kind of threat to health that alcoholic fatty liver disease does.

Low Carb Diets and Heartburn

One positive side effect that is often reported by people on very low carb diets is that their heartburn clears up entirely as soon as they cut out the carbs. That this effect is real was documented in a small study of eight obese people conducted by Dr. Westman's Atkins-funded team at Duke. (Austin, 2006)

The participants in this study were given 24-hr esophageal pH probe testing, once before beginning a ketogenic diet and again six days after they started it. The amount of time they spent with the pH

---

[12] You'll find a discussion of the problems with the HOMA calculation on page 110.

of their stomach acid less than 4 decreased from 5.1% to 2.5%. (The lower the pH the stronger the acid.)

The healing effect low carb dieting has on heartburn is often observed by people posting on online diet discussion boards. It persists as long as they stay on the diet and sometimes after they have raised their carbohydrate intake significantly. It is unknown whether this decrease in heartburn is caused by cutting back on carbohydrates or because traditional very low carb diets cut out all grains, which eliminates gluten.

It's possible that the gluten is what causes the heartburn, since the high carbohydrate gluten-free diets eaten by people diagnosed with celiac disease also eliminate heartburn. (Nachman, 2011) If this is the case, eating commercially prepared foods marketed as "low carb" that contain gluten, like some "low carb" tortillas may undo this effect.

Points to Remember from This Chapter:

1. Heavier people lose more weight on low carb diets than lighter ones.

2. Common side effects of ketogenic diets include constipation, headache, bad breath, muscle cramps, diarrhea, general weakness, and rash. We'll discuss how to deal with these in Chapter 11.

3. Low carb diets do not cause significant problems with mood or cognition.

4. Ketogenic low carb diets are effective, but because they are so difficult for most people to stick to, it is important to consider what happens to people who abandon them.

5. When people continue to eat very high fat diets after raising their carbohydrates, their triglyceride and LDL levels rise in ways that may harm their health. Keeping fat intake high as carb intake rises also raises calories which can lead to a swift regain of lost weight. If you raise your carbs out of the low carb range, keeping your fat intake to 30% of all calories consumed will help to avoid these problems.

6. Low carb diets improve fasting insulin, fasting glucose, and post-meal blood sugars while people are eating them. But there is no evidence that they make permanent changes that persist after people end their diets.

7. Ketogenic low carb diets improve the blood sugars of people with diabetes with no relationship to how much weight they lose. But few people with diabetes can stick to them for very long, making less

stringent low carb diet containing less fat a better choice for many people with diabetes.

8. Diet alone is not enough to give some people with severe diabetes the normal blood sugars that will prevent them from suffering diabetic complications. Matching carb restriction with carefully chosen, properly prescribed medications is essential.

9. Ketogenic low carb diets may decrease levels of liver fat. But it is not clear if they do this because of some effect attributable to being in a ketogenic state or because they cause weight loss.

10. Very low carb diets appear to relieve heartburn, though it isn't clear if this is caused by limiting carbohydrates or by eliminating gluten.

Chapter 5
The Low Carb Diet and Hunger

We started our discussion of the low carb diet by explaining that blood sugars that go up and down like a rollercoaster cause the hunger that makes it so hard to diet. Many people find that a low carb diet that normalizes their blood sugars also stills this hunger. Now we'll look at what researchers have learned about how low carb diets affect hunger.

For an overview, we'll turn first to a research report drawing on data collected during the two-year low carb/low fat comparison study we discussed in Chapter 3, which tested participants for ketone levels. This report is titled, "Change in Food Cravings, Food Preferences, and Appetite During a Low-Carbohydrate and Low-Fat Diet." (Martin, 2011) It concluded that,

> The [Low Carb Diet] group reported being less bothered by hunger compared to the [Low Fat Diet] group. . . . Men had larger decreases in appetite ratings compared to women. Prescription of diets that promoted restriction of specific types of foods resulted in decreased cravings and preferences for the foods that were targeted for restriction. The results also indicate that the L[ow]C[arb]D[iet] group was less bothered by hunger compared to the L[ow]F[at]D[iet] group and that men had larger reductions in appetite compared to women.

This difference between men and women in how well the low carb diet controls their hunger may explain why most of the super-losers you encounter in the online diet community are male. It may also point to the strong impact that cycling female hormones have on appetite—an effect that is not eliminated by controlling blood sugar and which can ramp up hunger very strongly the week before menstruation.

But even though the low diet made people less hungry than the low fat diet in this study, 42% of the people eating the low carb diet dropped out before it ended, 16% of them before they had completed even 6 full months. Thirty-seven percent were no longer eating a ketogenic diet 3 months after starting their diets. So even if the low carb dieters were less hungry than the low fat dieters, they may still have been hungrier than people who weren't dieting at all, and over time this may have taken a toll.

Though factors other than hunger may explain why so many dieters raised their carbohydrate intake so quickly, it would be a mistake to completely dismiss the idea that changes in the hormones associated with hunger may have also played a role in undermining these dieters' dedication. Hunger is a complex phenomenon linked to a great number of hormones that interact with each other and with the brain. These interactions are very complex and not well understood, so you should be very wary of claims by diet gurus that *any* diet is effective because of the way it affects a specific hunger hormone.

When we look at how any diet affects a hunger hormone, two separate issues come up. One is how the makeup of a meal influences how hungry people feel after eating it. To study that researchers feed people meals containing different kinds of nutrients and take blood samples at intervals after they eat.

But the hormones that regulate hunger may change their behavior when people lose a lot of body fat. Death from starvation is high on the list of the things our brains worry about. So a diet that quells hunger in a person whose weight remains stable may no longer do so when that person has burned through enough stored body fat to make their ever-vigilant brain think they are in the midst of a long-lasting famine. To learn how diets change the behavior of hunger hormones after significant weight loss, researchers measure the levels of various hormones before and after people embark on long-term diets.

None of the large comparison studies we looked at in Chapter 3 measured how the low carb diet affected dieters' hunger hormones, but other smaller studies did. And what they've found paints a more complex picture of how the low carb diet alters hunger hormones, one that may help explain why the enthusiasm so common among new low carb dieters is so likely to fade out a few months after they begin their diets.

Leptin

Leptin was the first hunger hormone to be identified and possibly the best known. The discovery that mice lacking leptin ate constantly and stopped eating when they were given leptin raised hopes that supplementing with leptin could help overweight humans. But it turns out that most overweight humans have higher than normal levels of leptin and that obesity caused by leptin deficiency is profoundly rare in humans.

It also turns out that any diet that achieves weight loss will lower leptin. By the time an overweight person has lost 10% of their starting weight their leptin levels will have dropped dramatically. Leptin's job seems to be to tell the body that it's time to refill depleted fat stores. It is part of the exquisite system our bodies have evolved to keep us from dying in the next famine.

When leptin has dropped, people become more focused on food because of leptin's effect on the brain's reward center. (Science Daily: Reward) Because these lowered leptin levels that are caused by weight loss make it so tough for dieters to maintain their weight losses, very recent research has looked into whether injecting leptin may help make it easier for people who have lost a lot of weight to maintain that weight loss. One study concludes that it does. (Kissileff, 2012)

But before you head to the doctor asking for your leptin shot, you might want to know that more research needs to be done to make certain it's safe to replace the leptin that newly-slim dieters have lost. That's because the high leptin levels overweight dieters have *before* they lose weight turn out to correlate with high levels of CRP, a measure of inflammation. When CRP rises, platelets tend to clot aggressively and blood pressure also rises—all factors contributing to heart disease. (de Moraes, 2005)

Though scientists hoped this association might be due to the fact that the fat cells of very heavy people are often inflamed, rather than to their higher leptin levels, this turned out not to be the case. A carefully controlled study where human leptin was injected into thin, young women who were put on a 4-day fast suggested that it was, in fact, the leptin, not the fat, that was causing this increase in inflammatory markers.

The thin subjects who received the leptin injections during their fast developed significantly higher CRP, as well as increased platelet aggregation. Their serum levels of amyloid A, another factor related to inflammation, increased, too. (Canavan, 2005)

This suggests that it may be healthier for people whose weight loss has left them with lower leptin levels to live with those lowered levels, though the cost of doing that may be having to live with a brain chemistry that is continually urging them to take just one more bite.

Studies of how the low carb diets affects leptin come up with mixed results. A meta-analysis that combined data from seven small, very short studies of truly ketogenic diets was conducted by a team at the University of Connecticut that included Jeff Volek, another of the three authors of the new Atkins book. It found, "There were greater reductions in leptin after the VLCKD [Very Low Carb Diet] (-50%) than the low-fat diet (-17%). The ratio of leptin/total fat mass also decreased more after the VLCKD (-45%) than the low-fat diet (-21%)." (Volek, 2004)

But all the studies whose data was mixed together to produce this meta-analysis lasted only a short time and involved a small number of subjects, leaving open the question of how valid any result might that is derived by artificially blending this scanty data using the statistical tricks characteristic of meta-analyses.

And because so many other studies have shown that leptin declines in parallel with weight loss, it is difficult to attribute the steeper drop in leptin found in this meta-analysis to the composition of the diet. It is just as possible that the steeper drop was due to the more rapid weight loss the low carb dieters experienced in the early weeks of their diets.

Long-term Results Yield Another Cautionary Tale

A study that provided follow-up to a short, 6-month low carb/low fat comparison study gives more insight into what happens to leptin over the long term. The study is titled, "The effects of a low-carbohydrate versus low-fat diet on adipocytokines in severely obese adults: three-year follow-up of a randomized trial." (Cardillo, 2006)

In the original study, the subjects in the low carb arm of the study ate a ketogenic diet for about 6 months, and their leptin levels dropped lower than those of a group of low fat dieters. This echoes Volek's results. But these researchers didn't stop there. Three years later they brought back a subset of the original subjects and examined them again.

What they found was disturbing. Just as happened to the backsliding low carb dieters in the other study we discussed in Chapter 4, the dieters in this study also abandoned their low carb diets after the study was over. Though they were eating less calories each day and 12% less carbohydrate than they had been eaten before they started their low carb diets, their carbohydrate intake worked out to an average of 187 grams of carbohydrate a day, a level that no one would consider "low carb."

But these erstwhile low carb dieters had continued to eat a high fat diet, so three years after starting their diets they were taking in 10% more fat than they had been eating before they started dieting. This extra fat did not negatively impact their weight maintenance when compared to that of the low fat dieters, because the erstwhile low carb dieters had also cut down on their calories. So over the three years, the low carb and low fat diet groups both maintained the same unimpressive weight loss—an average of 9 pounds in a group whose average BMI had started out at 43. But the increased fat intake of the erstwhile low carb dieters did have a negative impact on other measures of health.

It undid whatever benefits the ketogenic diet had made in their fasting insulin levels. One third of both diet groups started their diets with diagnoses of Type 2 diabetes. Three years after they had stopped eating their 6 month-long low carb diet, the erstwhile low carb dieters' average fasting blood glucose and insulin levels had risen *above* where they had been before the study started, though the low fat dieters had maintained small improvements in theirs.

The impact on leptin was even worse. While they had been dieting, the low carb dieters' average leptin level had dropped much lower than that of the low fat dieters. But 3 years later, the erstwhile low carb dieters' leptin levels were *higher* than they had been at the study's start, though the erstwhile low fat dieters' leptin had continued to drop and was lower than it had been 6 months into their diet.

Once again, the conclusion here is that whatever short-term changes a low carb diet makes in leptin and other metabolic parameters, when dieters go back to eating carbs and keep eating *more* fat than they used to eat, bad things happen. Eating extra fat raises their leptin levels, but even if this may make them less hungry, it's not healthy.

These very heavy, erstwhile low carb dieters had also started their diets with the very high leptin levels characteristic of people with high BMIs. Their leptin levels had started out, on average, more than twice as high as the leptin levels of the thin young women studied in the Canavan study we discussed above.

They ended up with leptin levels that, on average, were about 10% higher than those they had started with. So the end result of their flirtation with low carb dieting was to teach them a very bad habit—eating more fat along with a lot of carbs—that enhanced their chances of developing the inflammation and tendency to blood clots associated with very high leptin levels. This raised their likelihood of getting heart disease.

Does Intermittent Fasting Keep Leptin from Dropping?

Some low carb aficionados will tell you that you can avoid lowering your leptin levels by fasting every other day. There is little research validating this approach in humans, and what there is involves very small sample sizes. But the research we have contradicts this theory.

One study describes an eight week-long diet that used alternate day fasting. Its dieters consumed only 500 calories on their fasting days. Despite this alternate day fasting, these dieters experienced the same significantly lower leptin levels that regular dieters experience after they spent 8 weeks on their diets.

Just as was the case with other diets, the amount that an individual's leptin dropped turned out to relate entirely to how much weight and fat they had lost. This suggests that there is no easy way to fool a metabolism shaped by millions of years of surviving an environment where starvation, not obesity is the most dangerous threat. Leptin's job is to get us replenishing our fat stores after a period of starvation, and it does it very well. (Bhutani, 2010)

Ghrelin

Though leptin will make you hungrier when your fat mass has shrunk and doesn't seem to care about what you've done to your blood sugar levels, another important hunger hormone does, and the way it works may help explain why many of us find that blood sugar spikes after meals make us hungry and contribute to the overeating that causes obesity.

Ghrelin is a hormone produced in the stomach and pancreas that has been linked to feelings of hunger. In normal people, the higher the ghrelin level, the more hunger. Many studies have found that ghrelin levels are lower in obese people, but even so, they rise and fall after meals in obese people in exactly the same pattern found in normal people.

A comprehensive published review of ghrelin research tells us that women have higher ghrelin levels than men at all times. But women's ghrelin levels rise even more—to a level 3-fold higher than men's— during the late follicular stage of their menstrual cycle. This may help explain the rise in appetite that so many women experience at they approach their periods. Ghrelin levels also drop in the elderly which may have something to do with why they often lose their appetites. (Yin, 2009)

Almost as soon as a normal person eats a high carbohydrate meal they experience a release of insulin, and when this happens, their ghrelin level, which is highest before a meal, drops to half its starting level. This happens by 20 minutes after the start of the meal, and when it does, it decreases the normal person's feeling of hunger. This is why when normal people eat high carbohydrate meals, they don't feel hungry afterwards.

Most interestingly, though you will often read in diet books that fat is more satisfying than protein, ghrelin levels decline more after eating *protein* than they do after eating fat. This suggests that eating protein may do a better job of eliminating the hunger symptoms caused by ghrelin than eating fat. (Foster-Schubert, 2008)

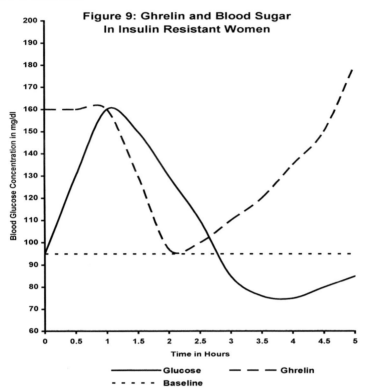

Figure 9: Ghrelin and Blood Sugar In Insulin Resistant Women

But studies also document that when insulin resistant people with mildly elevated blood sugars eat a high carbohydrate meal, their ghrelin, after an initial drop, rebounds very strongly only a few hours after that meal. This makes them hungrier than they were before they ate.

When the blood sugar, insulin, and ghrelin levels of these insulin resistant people are sampled at various times after their meal, their blood sugar values remain within the range doctors consider normal. They never drop anywhere near the level doctors label hypoglycemia—a level known to cause hunger. But even so, their blood sugars drop well below their *usual* fasting level. And this drop, even though it occurs entirely within the normal range, makes their ghrelin rise until it is higher than it was before their meal.

This may provide a scientific basis for explaining why people with diabetes who use blood sugar meters often note that steep drops in blood sugar, even those that don't push their blood sugar into the hypoglycemic range, provoke relentless hunger.

You can see this graphed in Figure 9 above. This graph uses data published in a study of insulin resistant women with PCOS who were fed different substances and given a glucose tolerance test.[13] (Kasim-Karakas, 2007)

Note that this rebound in ghrelin levels only appears to happen when people eat enough carbohydrate to raise their blood sugar into the upper part of the range doctors consider normal, which we explained is really abnormal, back in Chapter 1.

The same study of women with PCOS documented a very different pattern of ghrelin production when these same women were fed a meal that contained nothing but 75 grams of protein. The protein meal still made their insulin rise to a level much higher than it would in normal people. A normal person's insulin concentration tends to be around 18 µIU/dl 2 hours after they take a glucose challenge and considerably lower after a protein challenge. (Shaham, 2008) But these women's insulin levels rose to an average of 80 µIU/dl two hours after they consumed their high protein meal. Even so, their ghrelin responded very differently to the low protein meal than it had to the high carbohydrate one.

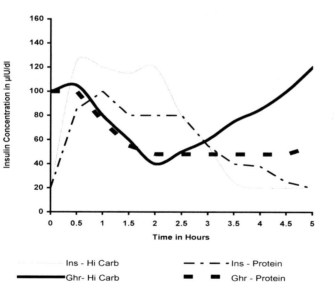

Figure 10: Ghrelin and Insulin In Insulin Resistant Women Fed All Carb and All Protein Meals

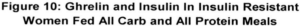

---

[13] Polycystic Ovary Syndrome is a condition in which women experience an abnormal hormonal balance that leads them to develop small cysts on their ovaries, abnormal hair growth, irregular or missing periods, and high levels of testosterone. Many, though not all, women with PCOS are extremely insulin resistant.

As you can see in figure 10 on page 85, the protein meal kept their blood sugar completely flat, and without that drop and rebound caused by eating carbohydrate, their ghrelin remained low after the protein meal, barely rising over the next four hours. That pattern of ghrelin secretion should prevent hunger, and the fact that ghrelin levels stay flat even when people secrete abnormally high amounts of insulin after eating a protein meal contradicts the oft repeated but poorly supported argument that it is surging insulin, not glucose, that causes hunger.

I have not been able to find much useful research that provides data showing whether this flattening effect on the hunger hormone ghrelin, which we see after people eat one very low carb protein meal, continues as people eat a low carb diet for more than a meal or two.

There is one study in which 20 dieters were supposed to eat a self-selected South Beach Diet that was 10% carbohydrate for 2 weeks. Then they were supposed to switch to eating a South Beach diet that was 27% carbohydrate for the next ten weeks. This 27% carbohydrate diet was so low in calories that the 27% that was supplied by carbs only worked out to 96 grams a day.

These dieters' *fasting* ghrelin levels slowly rose throughout the study but no measurement was made of their post-meal levels. The researchers noted that this correlated with "increased subjective reports of hunger." This study can't answer the question of whether the rise in ghrelin was caused by carbohydrate restriction, calorie restriction, weight loss or some combination of all three. (Haye, 2007)

Another small study of 10 men with Type 2 diabetes who ate a ketogenic diet for two weeks measured their ghrelin levels throughout the day before and after they ate the diet. It found that for the group as a whole, the average ghrelin level rose slightly after two weeks on the diet.

This study also analyzed the total amount of ghrelin secreted by individual subjects. It found that it rose in almost all the individuals studied, but a graph depicting the Area Under the Curve for ghrelin for individual study subjects shows that the higher the individual's ghrelin levels were to start with, the more they rose after two weeks on the diet. (Boden, 2005)

A study by Volek's team at the University of Connecticut reports a result that contradicted the one in the previous study. In this one, a small number of men eating a carbohydrate-restricted diet for 12 weeks did not experience a rise in their ghrelin levels. (Ratliff, 2009)

We have no way of knowing why these two studies came up with different findings. But since these studies only enrolled a small number of participants, this kind of variation is to be expected. In small studies, the characteristics of a few individuals can skew the data for the group. It takes more participants to provide a more trustworthy conclusion.

Both these studies were also very short. Twelve weeks is well within the honeymoon phase of ketogenic dieting. We would need to see what happens to ghrelin after a year or two on the diet before drawing any conclusions. Let's hope future research investigates this.

Peptide YY

Studies also strongly associate another gut hormone with hunger: Peptide YY (PYY). PYY is a protein secreted both in the lining of the digestive tract and, in lesser amounts, in the brain and pancreas. Like most peptides it has more than one function, but one of the things it does is to slow the rate at which the stomach empties. When your stomach doesn't empty you feel full, sometimes uncomfortably so, and, sure enough, giving people infusions of extra PYY cuts way back on how much they eat when they are provided with an "all you can eat" buffet. Giving people too much PYY makes them nauseated to the point where they may vomit. (Batterham, 2003)

When normal people eat high carbohydrate meals, the concentration of PYY in their bloodstream rises, making them feel full and shutting down hunger. But a study found that this is not the case with severely overweight young teens. This study was investigating the behavior of PYY in three groups of teens, one normal, one anorectic, and one obese. It found that PYY's normal effect—creating a feeling of fullness—was "blunted" in the obese girls. When *they* ate carbohydrates, the level of PYY in their bloodstreams, which had started out higher than that of the normal weight girls, barely rose. The same appears to be the case with obese adults, too. The teen study found no relationship between the changes the girls experienced in their blood sugar levels, insulin levels, and their PYY levels during their meal. (Stock, 2005)

So what happens to PYY levels when you put these obese people who don't properly release PYY on a very low carbohydrate diet? Here is where things get interesting. One study found that after eating a low carb diet for a week, the levels of PYY in a group of obese low carb dieters were one and a half times higher than those of a similar group of dieters eating a low fat diet. This suggests that they would have felt much fuller. (Essah, 2007)

But this effect was short-lived. After eight weeks on their diets, the people eating low carb diets no longer had higher levels of PYY in their bloodstream than the low fat dieters. This was true, even though as a group the low carb dieters had lost 10 more pounds on average than the low fat dieters, which strongly suggests that they had indeed been eating ketogenic diets—and that burnt off glycogen explained the much greater weight loss they achieved over a short period of time.

At the eight week point, both groups of dieters saw, on average, a 9% drop in this hunger-quenching hormone, with a trend toward the people who had lost the most weight experiencing the largest drop. So it is possible that weight loss—or decreasing the volume of food that goes into the stomach—has a stronger impact on PYY than diet composition.

There are several other hormones that are known to have an effect on hunger including amylin, a hormone secreted along with insulin, which affects stomach emptying, and the incretin hormones GIP and GLP-1. Byetta, a diabetes drug which supplies a long-acting artificial form of GLP-1, stimulates insulin production while also slowing stomach emptying. It produces dramatic weight losses in one third of the people who take it. However, Byetta works best if people eat enough carbohydrate to raise their blood sugar to the 120 mg/dl level where a burst of insulin secretion is triggered. I could not find any human research that examines what effects, if any, ketogenic or low carb diets may have on GIP and GLP-1.

Overall, the message that emerges from studies of all these hunger-related hormones is that, whatever the short term effect may be of cutting back on carbs, as a diet continues and weight loss occurs, hunger hormones alter in ways that make people hungrier, more interested in food, and less likely to feel full. This means that anyone embarking on a diet, no matter what its nutrient composition must accept that any significant weight loss will increase their interest in food, and eventually may cause some hunger that won't be entirely erased by flattening their blood sugar.

This may partially explain why even in groups of highly motivated dieters, weight loss slows down or stops roughly 6 months after they've started their low carb diets.

MSG

Though it isn't a hunger hormone, Monosodium glutamate (MSG) is a chemical present in much of the food we eat which has a strong impact on hunger. It is added to many prepared and restaurant foods and has long been known to cause overeating and weight gain. Because it is so often present in processed foods, especially meats, many low carb dieters unwittingly raise their intake of this chemical when they switch to low carb diets and eat more processed and fast food meats.

Rodent research has found that eating MSG leads to an increase in insulin resistance that happens because cells lose their glucose receptors. (de Carvalho, 2002) MSG also decreases blood ketone levels in sheep and raises their blood sugars. (Thompson, 1968).

But there is a surprising lack of published research investigating whether MSG has the same effects on humans. The most compelling evidence that it does emerges from a study published in 2008 by scientists at the University of North Carolina who not only documented that eating MSG makes people fat, but that eating MSG causes weight gain *independent* of how much a person eats or how much they exercise.

The study was conducted in China among peasants eating a traditional home-cooked diet that was without any other additives except for MSG, which has long been a part of the traditional Chinese diet. (He, 2008)

The researchers followed more than 750 Chinese men and women, aged between 40 and 59, in three rural villages in north and south China. The majority of study participants prepared their meals at home without commercially processed foods. About 82% of the participants used MSG in their food.

The researchers broke those who used MSG into three groups, based on the amount of MSG they used. They found that the third who used the most MSG were nearly *three times* more likely to be overweight than non-users. The prevalence of overweight was significantly higher in MSG users than in non-users even after the researchers controlled for physical activity, total calorie intake, and other possible explanations for the differences in their body mass.

MSG is produced by fermenting protein-rich foods, which is why it occurs naturally in soy sauce. But most of our exposure comes from processed and restaurant foods where it's added as a flavor enhancer. Many fast food and chain restaurants add MSG to their meats, perhaps to increase their patrons' appetites.

Because food manufacturers know that many people consider MSG to be unhealthy, labels hide it by using various legally-allowed pseudonyms including: natural flavoring, textured protein, hydrolyzed protein, yeast extract, glutamate, glutamic acid, calcium caseinate, hydrolyzed corn gluten, monopotassium glutamate, sodium caseinate, yeast nutrient, yeast food, natrium glutamate, and autolyzed yeast.

Points to Remember from This Chapter:

1. Lowered leptin levels make us obsess about food, but high leptin levels are bad for our health. Leptin levels appear to drop in response to weight loss caused by any diet, including low carb diets.

2. Eating more fat after raising your carbohydrate intake can raise leptin to higher levels than you started with and enhance your likelihood of developing heart disease.

3. Ghrelin is the hunger hormone most closely tied to blood sugar levels and the way it responds to blood sugar fluctuations may explain why some people get hungry after eating high carb meals that cause a blood sugar spike. Ghrelin rises on some low carb diets and stays constant on others, but there is not enough data to make any claims about the ability of the low carb diet to control levels of this hormone, especially over long term.

4. Peptide YY affects how full we feel, but though a low carb diet may lower it temporarily, like the other hunger hormones, PYY rises as diets continue and people lose weight.

5. MSG increases insulin resistance and causes weight gain independent of what people eat. Low carb dieters should be careful to avoid eating processed and fast food meats that are laced with it.

Chapter 6

Low Carb Controversies

The research we've just reviewed should have answered many of your questions about the safety and efficacy of low carb diets. But because any mention of the low carb diet still evokes strong emotional responses from friends, relatives, and doctors, we'll look next at some of the more controversial claims you're likely to hear once you embark on a low carb diet and examine the peer-reviewed research that addresses these claims.

Does the Low Carb Diet Raise Cholesterol and Cause Heart Attacks?

We've already learned that every study that compared low carb diets to other diets found that the low carb diets improved many of the health parameters used to evaluate the risk of heart disease as long as people stuck to them. While it's true that low carb diets do raise LDL levels more than other diets, the changes they make to triglycerides and HDL suggest that LDL becomes lighter and fluffier, which makes it less likely to turn into artery-clogging plaque. The low carb diet also lowers blood pressure, CRP, fasting glucose and insulin, all of which point to it decreasing the risk of developing cardiovascular disease.

As we've also seen, the health problems associated with the low carb diet occur only when people *abandon* it while continuing to eat the large amounts of fat that are only healthy when consumed in the absence of carbohydrate.

Even so, after you've been eating a low carb diet for a few months, your doctor is likely to tell you your LDL has gone up and to order you to take a cholesterol-lowering statin drug. Should you take it? The bestselling diet books assure you this high LDL isn't a problem, but they do a poor job of explaining how you can determine if this is really true for you. Given how serious the threat of heart attack is, you need more than the assurance of some distant diet doctor who has never examined you that it's safe to ignore the advice of your personal doctor.

To give you the tools you need to make an informed decision, we'll start by reviewing what science has learned about how well the commonly applied blood tests predict cardiovascular events—the term doctors use to refer to heart attacks, stroke, and the presence of arteries clogged so severely they require stenting.

LDL Does Not Predict Heart Attacks

Despite the public's widespread belief that high cholesterol causes heart attacks, research on this topic paints a more complex picture. The title of a review published in 1998 sums this up nicely: "Fifty percent of patients with coronary artery disease do not have any of the conventional risk factors." (Futterman, 1998) In fact, this study turns out to have underestimated what a poor job cholesterol does at predicting heart attacks.

A later study, published in 2009, which analyzed data from 136,905 Americans hospitalized for heart attacks between 2000 and 2006, found that roughly 72% had what doctors consider to be completely normal LDL—a concentration below 130 mg/dl—when they were tested at the hospital after admission for a heart attack. A further 17.6% had *low* LDL levels—below 70 mg/dl. (Sachdeva, 2009)

Though these findings should have made a reasonable person question whether LDL concentrations could be used to predict cardiac health, the authors of the 2009 study argued their findings only meant that LDL levels need to be lowered even more.

This is a tribute to the brainwashing job done by the companies that sell expensive statin drugs. They have sold doctors on the idea that LDL levels can predict heart attacks because that is what their statin drugs do: lower LDL. Statins have no effect on the *other* lipid fractions that some very high quality epidemiological research has found to be much better indicators of cardiac health.

The drug companies can spend billions of dollars on "education" telling doctors that high LDL is all they should worry about because the statin drugs are obscenely profitable. In 2010, just two of the many statin drugs available, Lipitor and Crestor, earned their manufacturers 16.39 billion dollars. (Larkin, 2011)

What the Framingham Data Says About LDL

As early as 1996, analysis of the data collected by The Framingham Study, which tracked a large number of people for 35 years, revealed that LDL and total cholesterol don't reliably predict heart attacks. The Framingham Study identified two other cholesterol measurements that were slightly more reliable: One is the ratio of total cholesterol to

HDL. The other is the concentration of plasma triglycerides. (Castelli), 1996) The Framingham data suggested that the risk of heart disease rises when the ratio of Total Cholesterol to HDL (TC/HDL), rises over 3 and when the concentration of fasting triglycerides in the bloodstream rises over 150 mg/dl.

Subsequent studies have suggested that as HDL drops and triglycerides rise, the amount of LDL that occurs in the form of small dense particles rises, too, and that it is these small dense particles that seep into the linings of arteries and cause the plaque that leads to heart attacks. As we mentioned earlier, the researchers who investigated what the low carb diet does to cholesterol pointed out that it raises HDL and lowers triglycerides in a way that suggests that LDL shifts toward the larger, fluffier, safer form—but only while you are actually eating a low carb diet. As we saw in the earlier research, once carbohydrates rise over 150 grams a day, the higher LDL caused by eating a high fat intake may very well be the kind that damages arteries.

To further complicate matters, it turns out that labs don't determine your LDL by actually measuring it. Instead they measure your total cholesterol, HDL, and triglycerides and then calculate your LDL level by applying a formula called the Friedwald equation. The formula is heavily based on your triglyceride level. Though many doctors know that the Friedwald equation is inaccurate when triglycerides are higher than 400 mg/dl, few realize that it is *also* inaccurate when triglycerides fall into the *lower* part of the normal range—which is exactly where they will fall when you cut the carbs out of your diet. This may be another reason why cutting carbs raises LDL test results.

Unfortunately, the study documenting this effect was published in a very low impact journal, *Archives of Iranian Medicine*, so the finding has been completely ignored. (Ahmadi, 2008)You can find a calculator online which will apply the findings of this study to your own test results:

> http://homepages.slingshot.co.nz/~geoff36/LDL_mg.htm

Other studies have found that measuring something called ApoB is more predictive of heart disease than LDL, at least for some groups of people. ApoB is a protein found attached to LDL molecules so the more LDL molecules you have, the more ApoB you'll have. High levels of ApoB correlate better with the presence of clogged arteries than do LDL levels. For example one study found "Plasma apoB, but not LDL cholesterol, levels were associated with CAC [coronary artery calcification] scores in type 2 diabetic whites." (Martin, 2009)

But medical journals are packed with studies that advance the claims of dozens of different lipid ratios, subfractions and other cholesterol-related factors for predicting who will get a heart attack — studies that contradict each other and often fail to be confirmed by subsequent studies. The more you study the subject, the more you'll come to see that no measurement related to lipids provides a hard and fast guide to heart attack risk.

Blood Sugar Tests *Do* Predict Heart Attacks

This uncertainty vanishes when we turn to a completely different body of research. Though few doctors know this, and statin-selling drug reps are not about to mention it, there are several *blood sugar tests* that reliably and reproducibly predict cardiac events far better than do any cholesterol tests.

This was first announced in 2004 with the publication of the results of a large-scale study called EPIC-Norfolk. What's particularly valuable about this study is that its designers weren't looking for the causes of heart disease. They were studying *cancer* and they were looking at blood sugar because of their belief that it might be related to cancer incidence, which turned out not to be the case. This made their finding that a blood sugar test, the A1C, predicted heart disease in people with supposedly normal blood sugar a shocker.

As we explained earlier, the A1C test estimates how high an individual's blood sugar has been over a period of about three months. What the EPIC-Norfolk study found was that "In men and women, the relationship between hemoglobin A1C and cardiovascular disease ... was continuous and significant throughout the whole distribution." This means, in plain English, that, as the A1C rose, the incidence of cardiovascular disease also rose.

What's more, they add,

> The relationship was apparent in persons without known diabetes. ... These relative risks were independent of age, body mass index, waist-to-hip ratio, systolic blood pressure, serum cholesterol concentration, cigarette smoking, and history of cardiovascular disease.

They also explain, "Persons with hemoglobin A1C concentrations less than 5% had the lowest rates of cardiovascular disease and mortality." That would correspond to an average blood sugar level of 97 mg/dl, which is *different* from a fasting level of 97 mg/dl because this average takes into account all the blood sugar spikes after meals. (Khaw, 2004)

This finding was validated by two different analyses of data collected by another large epidemiological study, The Atherosclerosis Risk in Communities Study. (Selvin, 2005 and Selvin, 2010)

These findings make it clear that the range doctors currently consider "normal" for the A1C, a range that goes up to 6.4%, is, in fact, far from normal, unless you define "normal" as meaning, "having two to three times the risk of cardiovascular disease," which is how much more risk a person with a 6.4% A1C has compared to one with a 5.0% A1C according to these studies.

One of these studies (Selvin, 2010) tracked 11,092 black or white adults who did not have a history of diabetes or cardiovascular disease for 15 years. It found no association between their *fasting blood sugars* and their risk of heart disease—which is significant, because the fasting blood sugar test is the *only* test most doctors give patients to see if they have abnormal blood sugars. But when it came to the A1C, it was another story. The A1C predicted cardiovascular risk, as shown by this table that maps risk ratios against various A1Cs, all of them in the range doctors consider normal:

A1C	Relative Risk of Cardiovascular Disease
5%:	0.96 (0.74-1.24) Roughly Normal
5% to < 5.5%:	1.00 (reference) Roughly Normal
5.5% to < 6%:	1.23 (1.07-1.41) Slightly higher risk
6% to < 6.5%:	1.78 (1.48-2.15) Up to twice as much risk

However, the A1C test, while useful to epidemiologists because it's cheap, measures what doctors call a surrogate marker." It doesn't actually measure your blood sugars but something else, which it uses to estimate them. Other research has proven that while the A1C is a useful test for studying large populations, individual A1C test results can be inaccurate for individuals whose red blood cells are longer lived than normal and for people with abnormal hemoglobin. (BS101: A1C)

Measuring actual post-meal blood sugars, though more expensive, turns out to give a more accurate prediction of heart attack risk. One study found that thickening in the arteries of people with diabetes correlated most closely not to their A1C results, but to how high their blood sugars rose after a meal eaten at home. (Esposito, 2008)

That this same relationship between post-meal blood sugar levels and cardiovascular disease is likely to hold true for people who do *not* have diabetes was confirmed by another study that found that people whose blood sugar rose over 155 mg/dl at one hour after the start of a glucose tolerance test had significantly higher measures of inflammation and of fibrinogen, a substance associated with clotting. Inflammation and abnormal clotting are both factors strongly associated with heart disease. (Bardini, 2009)

Now that you know that slightly abnormal blood sugar levels promote inflammation and abnormal clotting, it's easier to see why the Framingham Study found that triglyceride levels were most closely associated with heart disease risk. "Triglyceride" is just a fancy term for "animal fat," and it turns out that what raises the amount of fat floating around your bloodstream is how much carbohydrate you eat. This is because, as we explained earlier, after you digest carbohydrates, your liver transforms any unburned glucose into triglycerides, which it either stores within the liver itself, or dumps into the bloodstream for storage in fat cells.

With that in mind, we can see why eating a low carb diet might improve not only our cholesterol profiles, but also our likelihood of getting a heart attack. That's because people with high normal blood sugars who cut their carbs will stop having those damaging post-meal blood sugar spikes that thicken our arteries and inflame them. This suggests too, as the proponents of low carb diets claim, that the low carb diet lowers your risk of getting heart disease, even if it causes a rise in LDL, so long as your triglycerides drop.

But to this we should add that the low carb diet lowers your risk of heart attack as long as it makes your *blood sugars* drop to truly normal levels. If you are still getting blood sugars that rise over 155 mg/dl after you eat your low carb meal, your low carb diet has not eliminated your risk of having a heart attack.

One Size Does Not Fit All

This is where many of the diet books get things wrong. Because these books always make it sound as if there is some set amount of carbohydrate that, if you eat only that much, will eliminate your risk of heart disease. But the truth is, people vary greatly in the degree to which they can control their blood sugars. So there is no intake of carbs that will give everyone normal blood sugars.

Some people can eat 150 grams a day and see completely normal sugars. Some can eat 300 grams—and for these people, a low carb diet will be no more or less effective than any other diet that lowers calories. At the opposite extreme, there are people who can't get normal readings even if they eat less than 10 grams a day of carbohydrate.

They will need to rely on a few safe, well-test diabetes drugs doctors can prescribe to normalize their sugars.

That's because there are other factors involved in regulating blood sugar besides how much carbohydrate you eat. If your pancreas has suffered a mild, undetected, autoimmune attack, something which is becoming increasingly common in adults, or if you have damaged genes that impair your ability to secrete insulin, cutting carbs won't prevent you from having blood sugars that still rise over that 155 mg/dl level where inflammation and abnormal clotting become more common.

The Low Carb Diet is Not a Universal Heart Disease Cure

There are exceptions to every rule, and before we leave this discussion it's worth noting that there *are* a small number of people who have genetic flaws somewhere in their metabolisms that make it hard for them to metabolize fats properly. Some of them see their blood sugars *rise* when they eat low carb diets because they can't tolerate high fat diets. These people are rare but I've run into a few. And this points to how important it is to measure your own blood sugars the way you'll learn how to do in Chapter 9, before you embark on a diet that elimi-nate carbs and replaces them with fat.

People with other genetic flaws may continue to have very high cholesterol when they eat a very low carb diet, along with low HDL and triglycerides that are over 150 mg/dl. This suggests they may still be making small, dense, dangerous LDL, and for them a statin drug may be useful. The same is true for people who have been diagnosed with heart disease, and people who have evidence of inflammation in their arteries. The statin drugs would make sense for them, because they appear to be effective for reducing inflammation in the arteries.

Even if the low carb diet does, over time, reverse heart disease — something that has not been tested in any long-term study — given how few people stuck to their low carb diets for even a year in the stu-dies we examined, it would be premature to conclude that adopting a low carb diet is all you need to do to avoid a heart attack.

And because the research also shows very clearly that many people who give up on low carb diets boost their fat intake, while eating enough carbs to raise their blood sugars, your doctor's fears about your new diet may be valid. He may have seen that happen with other patients whose short-lived low carb diets *did* prove harmful in long term when they went on eating bacon and blue cheese dressing with their burger in its bun — and with a side order of fries.

If you can stick to your low carb diet and keep your blood sugars in the normal range for several years, you should lower your risk of heart disease and of quite a few other dangerous chronic conditions. But until you've proven that you can stick to a diet that normalizes your blood sugar for four or five years, you're not out of the woods, especially if you have symptoms, like high blood pressure, that point to the possibility that you have already developed early heart disease.

In that case, a statin might be worth considering. This is particularly true if you have a serious family history of heart attack or if tests reveal that your blood is full of factors that point to your having an inflammatory condition.

Gum Disease, Heart Disease, and Blood Sugar

There is quite a lot of evidence pointing to another significant cause of heart disease—gum disease. If your gums are inflamed, as is so often the case in middle age, your arteries are also likely to be inflamed and thickening. Smokers are more prone to developing gum disease than other people, and this may have something to do with their propensity to get heart attacks.

It turns out that the inflammation that accompanies gum disease, like all systemic inflammation, actually raises your blood sugar. Conversely, aggressive treatment of gum disease decreases arterial inflammation and thickening and lowers blood sugar. (Piconi, 2008) A meta-analysis published in 2010 found that treating gum disease in people with diabetes lowered their blood sugar significantly. (Teeuw, 2010)

Dr. Bernstein has been urging readers with diabetes to treat their gum disease aggressively for this reason, and there is no reason to think it isn't as much of a concern for people without diabetes, especially since it has long been known that gum disease raises cardiac-specific CRP in everyone and this c-s CRP may indicate a higher risk of developing heart disease.

If you don't already have gum disease, eating a lower carb diet will cut down on the amount of plaque that will build up on your teeth. This may keep you from developing gum disease, as it is this dental plaque that, over time, irritates your gums and invites infection. But if you already have established gum disease it may take more than a low carb diet to heal it. If you are told you have pockets in the gums around your teeth, don't take a "watchful waiting" approach. Find a good periodontist who will take an aggressive approach to eliminating your gum disease.

Does a Low Carb Diet Cause Kidney Damage?

The belief that high protein diets cause kidney damage is one reason why, for many years, doctors warned people that low carb diets would kill them, and why many doctors still warn patients away from them. None of the large studies we looked at found evidence of kidney damage in their subjects, including those involving people with diabetes. And, as we saw, these studies also showed that long-term adherence to even a modestly low carb diet improved blood pressure, which is important because high blood pressure is a major cause of kidney failure.

Though this did not emerge in the large diet comparison studies, because they excluded people who had any sign of early kidney damage, there is some evidence that the low carb diet not only doesn't promote kidney damage, but may also *reverse* kidney damage.

People who are able to normalize their blood sugars with a low carb diet often report that their kidney function recovers and that microalbumin disappears from their urine. A case report describing just this effect was published in 2006. (Nielsen, 2006)

A more recent animal study duplicated this result. Two months on a ketogenic diet completely eliminated markers of kidney disease in severely diabetic mice. (Poplawski, 2011)

Dr Bernstein, who has been living with insulin-dependent Type 1 diabetes since 1946, has been eating a ketogenic low carb diet since the 1970s. He tells us that he reversed his own, fairly advanced, diabetic kidney disease after eating a ketogenic low carb diet for several years. (Bernstein, 2007, pp xiv-xvii).

The reason your doctor may fear that a low carb diet will damage your kidneys is because it was long believed that it was eating large amounts of protein that caused kidney failure. However, this long-held belief has been called into question. A review of the published research on the topic of whether *low* protein diets actually help people with diabetes preserve kidney function, published in September of 2008, suggests they do *not* and that the ACE inhibitors and ARB drugs prescribed to lower blood pressure are just as effective. (Pan, 2008)

An editorial published along with Pan's findings points out that no research has been done to look into the impact of cutting carbs on the health of the diabetic kidney. (Kopple, 2008)

In his book, Dr. Bernstein explains that what appears to damage kidneys is sugar that bonds to proteins and triggers an inflammatory response, not the proteins themselves. He writes that, in animal models, lowering blood sugar to 100 mg/dl reverses that damage. (Bernstein, op cit, p. 450). Though the high protein diet *can* be dangerous in the presence of high blood sugars—those over 200 mg/dl.—Dr. Bernstein asserts that protein does not damage the kidney when blood sugars are in the normal range. His explanation of the mechanism by which high blood sugars damage the kidney is given in his book. It is more detailed than I can go into here, but is worth a look if this is an issue that concerns you or your doctor.

Are Low GI Foods Healthier than Cutting Carbs?

Back at the turn of the millennium, when the low carb diet had become very popular with the general public and people started cutting down dramatically on their intake of starches and sugars, mainstream nutritionists came up with a new rationale for prescribing a diet heavy in grains. Drawing on the work of Jennie Brand-Miller, an obscure Australian nutritionist, they proclaimed that some foods, though filled with carbohydrates, digest slowly and do not raise blood sugar, making them ideal not only for normal people but for people with diabetes.

Brand-Miller published a table giving the "Glycemic Index" (GI) values of a long list of foods. These values were determined by feeding them to groups of normal people and comparing how high they raised their blood sugars over 2 hours compared to pure glucose. High glycemic foods had values near 100. For example, boiled potatoes were given a GI value of 101. Foods with a glycemic index near 50 were considered very healthy. These included foods like oatmeal and whole wheat breads.

Not surprisingly, organizations like the Whole Grains Council, an industry-funded marketing group, jumped on this concept. Their www.wholegrainscouncil.org web site lists several studies arguing for the health benefits of eating low GI foods.

Many of the studies the grain industry cites—and may have funded—are deceptively designed. For example, some studies that claim that the low GI diet improves health and lowers blood sugars compare a diet rich in low GI foods with a Froot Loops diet—one made up entirely of sugar and starch. While it's true that whole rolled oats make for a healthier breakfast than do chips of sugar-infused starch colored with suspect coal tar derivatives, these studies never compare the impact their diet makes on blood sugar with the much more benign effect you'd see after eating a breakfast of ham and eggs.

What benefits low GI foods can claim derive from the fact that they take longer to digest, so the starch and sugar they contain dribble into the bloodstream producing a long, slow rise in blood sugar, that normal people's insulin can keep from turning into a spike. One of the studies The Whole Grain Council displays on their web site, as an example of the benefits to be had from eating low GI foods, reports that eating beans, whole barley, and rye kernels delays digestion and reduces how much food people eat at their next meal. (Higgins, 2012)

But whoever put together the Council's web site must not have read that whole study, because buried in its text is this gem:

> Oats and wholemeal bread, which contains processed whole grain material, do not provide a subsequent meal effect (Table 1). Indeed, processing, milling, and cooking at high temperatures may negate the subsequent meal effect or, in some instances, can even exacerbate postprandial glycemia [i.e. raise blood sugar a lot] at a subsequent meal.

And there in a nutshell is the problem with supposedly low GI foods. Many foods rank low on the glycemic index because they digest slowly, but as this study points out, all this means is that the rise in blood sugar it causes is *postponed*, not eliminated.

Foods sweetened with fructose rather than glucose will also rank low on the glycemic index, since fructose doesn't raise blood sugar but goes directly to the liver where, as we learned in Chapter 1, it is either converted into glycogen to be released as glucose later or turned into fat. That's why, Brand-Miller's table of GI values, which assigns white bread a GI value of 95, lists Coca Cola made with high fructose corn syrup as having the much lower GI of 63. Fresh orange juice has an even lower GI at 43, even though doctors routinely tell people who inject insulin to drink orange juice to raise their blood sugar if they start to develop dangerously low blood sugars. Brand-Miller's GI index also assigns bananas a GI of 46, despite the fact that a single banana containing 46 grams of carbohydrate—more than a Lender's Bagel—which, with its GI value of 72, Brand-Miller considers a far better choice than white bread. (Foster-Powell, 2002)

As comforting as these figures might be to the Coca Cola Company and purveyors of bagels everywhere, it turns out that the GI tables one team of nutritionists comes up with don't match those published by other nutritionists. That's because if you feed two different groups of people the same food, you will often get a different GI value. Researchers who embrace the GI theory really stretch to explain why this happens, because non-reproducible results usually mean death for a scientific theory. But nutritionists don't let non-reproducible results stop them when those results seem to confirm a strongly held belief, no matter how unscientific—especially nutritionists desperate for anything that could help them ignore the growing number of studies suggesting that the ultra low fat diets they have been promoting for the past two generations have been harming people with abnormally high blood sugars.

The other huge problem with the Glycemic Index is that it tells you only what foods do to the blood sugar of a *normal* person two hours after they eat the food. If your blood sugar is not normal, because your insulin doesn't work very well, your blood sugar may rise much higher than the glycemic index would predict. And the glycemic index also fails to tell you what a food will do to your blood sugar three or four hours after you eat it.

The highly resistant starch in dried pasta can take 4 or 5 hours to digest, but when it does, every gram of carbohydrate in that pasta turns into glucose and hits your bloodstream. Pasta may not create a sharp peak in your blood sugar, because the glucose releases so slowly, but it does require insulin for processing, which makes that much less insulin available to cover other foods—which is why, as the article we cited above explains, these low GI foods can raise blood sugar at the *next* meal, or, if you eat them at dinner, raise your fasting blood sugar the next morning.

Because fat also slows digestion, high carb foods that contain a lot of fat like pizza can also give deceptively low readings 2 hours after eating, which gives them low GIs. A Harvard Medical School web site lists "Pizza, Super Supreme (Pizza Hut)" as having a GI of 36 (Harvard Health Publications: GI) which is almost half the GI value of 58 given for "50% cracked wheat kernel bread," though nutritionists conveniently ignore this and never recommend that you eat a diet of "healthy" Super Supreme pizza.

Alas, for those of us who wish they would, every gram of carb in the crust of that pizza will turn into glucose eventually, and when it does it will go into your bloodstream. The combination of fat and carbohydrate, eaten together is not good for your arteries, and as we saw earlier, eating fat and carbohydrate together can get people into metabolic trouble.

If your blood sugar is only mildly abnormal, you may get better blood sugars eating low GI foods, especially those like beans, lentils, and unmilled whole grains like wheat berries and rye kernels. People whose blood sugar is only mildly abnormal, though they no longer secrete a strong burst of insulin at the beginning of a meal, usually have the ability to secrete enough insulin over the first hour after eating to dispose of the glucose produced by slow-digesting foods which will keep it from rising to unhealthy levels. For them, slow carbs do have an advantage and may be a reasonable dietary choice. To determine if this is true for you, you will have to test your blood sugar with a blood sugar meter after eating meals rich in low GI foods. Be sure to test them after that 2 hour period is over, too, to make sure that the rise in blood sugar they may cause isn't just being delayed.

Once grains have been milled into flour, all bets are off. A European study that fed three different whole grain breads to people with diabetes concluded that they raised blood sugar by the same amount as white bread. (Mesci, 2008)

Does a Low Carb Diet Make You More Insulin Resistant?

A doctor may tell you that eating a low carb diet will worsen your insulin resistance and that if you go off your low carb diet you will gain more weight than you would have, had you eaten a different kind of diet.

Even some of the doctors who write low carb diet books hint at this, warning that if you ever go off the diet, you'll gain back a lot more weight than you started out with. This may motivate some people to stay on the diet, but there is no evidence that it is true.

As we've seen, the studies do make it clear that some people who go off their low carb diets *do* end up gaining weight faster than those who eat a low fat diet, but the explanation of why this happens has nothing to do with any increase in their insulin resistance. Their speedy weight gain is largely due to the extra calories they are eating when they keep their intake of fat high even after adding in a lot more calories from carbs. Eating an additional 200 calories a day over what you're burning will pack 2 pounds on you every month.

It's also possible, as we saw in Chapter 2, that if you have drained your liver's supply of glycogen, when you go back to a nonketogenic diet you will store more glycogen in your liver than you did before, which would increase your weight, too, though we have no data to tell us if this would be a permanent change or not.

But the main reason some doctors believe that people who eat low carb diets become more insulin resistant is that people will see higher blood sugars when given glucose tolerance tests while they are eating a ketogenic diet.

These higher readings aren't caused by any change in how their bodies respond to insulin. They're caused by the down-regulation of several enzymes needed to burn glucose. (McDonald, 1998, p. 72) Since your body has switched to burning fats, most tissues don't need those enzymes and will switch to making the ones used to burn fat instead.

Once you raise your carbohydrate intake and switch your cells back to burning glucose, your body will rapidly get back to producing those needed enzymes. According to the sources cited by Lyle McDonald, once these enzymes have been downregulated, it will take roughly 5 hours for the liver to up regulate them again, and between 24 and 48 hours for your muscles to do the same.

This is why, if you must take a glucose tolerance test while eating a ketogenic low carb diet, you should eat 150 grams of carbs for three days before taking the test to make sure you have the enzymes needed to process glucose. Otherwise you may end up with a misleadingly high test result.

Do Atkins Diets Kill People?

A favorite argument of those who would like to frighten you away from eating a ketogenic diet is that they have proved fatal to otherwise healthy people. A careful scan of the evidence turns up a grand total of one research report of a teen who died while eating what is described as "a low-carbohydrate/high-protein, calorie-restricted dietary regimen that she had initiated on her own." She died of an abnormal electrolyte balance which is the kind of diet-related death that most often occurs when people eat badly designed starvation diets. (Stevens, 2002)

A starvation diet is defined as a diet that provides 300 to 500 calories a day. Very low calorie diets of all kinds, including a commercial "high protein" starvation diet popular in the 1970s, can cause fatal arrhythmias because they don't supply enough protein to maintain the heart muscle. Such diets can also severely unbalance your electrolytes, which can cause heartbeat abnormalities. Though they are sometimes used by doctors running obesity clinics, they require careful supervision, supplementation, and continual monitoring of blood mineral levels. Doing them on your own *is* dangerous.

But that said, you are much more likely to be struck by lightning than to die as a result of eating a low carb diet. There is only one such published case report linking a low carb diet to a death, though hundreds of thousands of people, if not millions, have tried low carb diets over the past decades.

Rare cases have also been reported of deaths in children who were eating the extreme ketogenic diets used to control epilepsy. They died of irregular heart beats. These deaths were attributed to selenium deficiency. (Bank, 2008) However, the ketogenic diet fed to children with epilepsy is lower in carbohydrates than an Atkins-style low carb diet, so low that it must be eaten under the close supervision of a nutritionist. Until recently, the epilepsy ketogenic diet also severely restricted fluids.

Other, less well-documented cases are often cited by scaremongers including one report of man who died of a heart attack while eating a low carb diet. In fact, several of the large research studies we cited in Chapter 3 reported that a participant in the low carb study group died or had a "cardiac event" during the 2 to 4 years the study lasted. However, deaths and cardiac events were also reported in the other arms of these studies where people were eating high carb diets. Most significantly, in the longer studies where such deaths occurred, more people died of heart ailments in the groups who were eating the *high* carb diets than in the groups eating the low carb diets.

Does this mean that all dieting is dangerous? No. Being seriously overweight is dangerous, and the dieters in these medical diet studies are almost always very overweight. Many may have already developed early, undetected, heart disease before they started their diets, unrelated to what they were eating during the study.

What's really disturbing is how often I hear from people who tell me that the same doctors who warn them that low carb diets are dangerous urge them to have Weight Loss Surgery (WLS). This, despite the fact that NPR reported in 2006 that one out of every 200 patients who have weight loss surgery die as a result of the surgery. The NPR story claimed that "more than 150,000" Americans every year have WLS surgery, which implies that 750 people die *each year* as a "side effect" of weight loss surgery. (Neighmond, 2006)

This statistic is confirmed by the statistics you can find on a surgeon-written web page which presents the death rates for different WLS techniques as reported by various studies. They range from 1.5 per thousand to 9 per thousand. (Bariatric Surgery Source)

You may also be told that WLS will normalize your blood sugar, a claim that is unsupported by the evidence advanced by its proponents — all of whom have a financial stake in selling the surgery or devices used in the surgery. When WLS lowers blood sugar, it does so because it makes it impossible for people to eat more than a tiny amount of carbohydrate without vomiting. That, of course, means that any "dangers" associated with the low carb diet would apply equally to WLS, since the surgery, in effect, forces people to eat very low carb diets whether they want to or not. You can achieve the same blood-sugar-lowering effect without amputating portions of your stomach and risking death or a lifetime of irreversible malnutrition. (BS101: WLS)

The media attention given to two cases of deaths supposedly associated with the Atkins diet was fueled by activists from a PETA-associated group, the deceptively named "Physicians Committee for

Responsible Medicine." (PCRM) PETA is an animal-rights group that campaigns tirelessly to convince everyone to eat a vegan diet. They uses scare tactics to try to frighten people away from eating meat and have a very active PR wing that orchestrates letter writing campaigns where people send letters to local newspapers all over the country—all featuring the identical wording—that make unsupported claims about how dangerous it is to eat meat.

PCRM vegan crusaders claim that Dr. Atkins himself died of a heart attack, advancing this as proof that his diet is dangerous. The Snopes web site gives a good explanation for what is actually known about Dr. Atkins' death. It states that he died of a fall.

The news media spread a story originating from PCRM that claimed that the New York City medical examiner had reported that the 72 year old Atkins had had a heart attack and was obese at the time of his death. This information had been provided to reporters by PCRM activists who, if they had obtained the medical examiner's report did so fraudulently, as it is illegal to release that kind of report to anyone but the patient's treating physician.

When questioned, the New York Medical examiner would state only that Dr. Atkins had died of a fall. After the PETA propagandists told the media that Dr. Atkins was obese at the time of his death, his wife released his death certificate and medical records. They showed that the 6 foot tall Dr. Atkins weighed 195 lbs upon his admission to the hospital after his fall. The subsequent weight gain noted on his death certificate was the result of the fluids he was treated with while in the coma caused by his fall. (Snopes: Atkins)

Points to Remember from This Chapter:

1. Low carbohydrate diets, when people stick with them, improve the one metabolic factor that has been tightly linked to heart disease risk: blood sugar.

2. A1C and blood sugar levels tested 1 hour after eating are far more predictive of heart attack risk than are any measures of cholesterol, possibly because lowering blood sugar improves triglycerides, which are among the lipids that have the best predictive value for heart disease.

3. Because so few people stick to low carb diets, you should not rely on a new low carb diet to protect you against heart disease until you have been on it for many years. People with strong risk factors for heart disease may benefit from taking statins.

4. High protein diets do not cause kidney disease. Low carb diets may reverse kidney disease over time by removing the glucose that bonds to proteins and causes them to become inflammatory.

5. Low GI foods are only beneficial if your blood sugar is truly normal after eating them, which is not the case for most people who have abnormal blood sugars. Milled flour, no matter whether it is "whole grain" or not, raises blood sugar as much as white flour.

6. Low carb diets do not make people more insulin resistant, nor do people gain more weight when they stop eating low carb diets if they don't keep eating high levels of additional fat.

7. The very few deaths attributed to low carb diets do not appear to have been caused by anything related to cutting down on carbohydrates. The low carb diet is far safer than Weight Loss Surgery, which has a very troubling death rate associated with it. Contrary to the claims of those with a financial stake in Weight Loss Surgery, it does not reverse or cure diabetes. Any benefits it has re blood sugar come from the fact that it makes it impossible for people to eat large quantities of carbohydrate.

Chapter 7

Low Carb Claims

In the previous chapter we took a hard look at the arguments advanced by those who will warn you about possible dangers associated with the low carb diet. In this chapter we'll give equal scrutiny to some of the claims made by enthusiastic proponents of the diet.

Do Ketogenic Diets Have a "Metabolic Advantage"?

Dr. Atkins' insistence that the ketogenic diet he'd branded with his name provides a "metabolic advantage" and his claim that dieters on his diet could eat "luxuriously" and still lose weight are another, ongoing source of controversy about the low carb diet.

We learned in Chapter 3 that one of the large comparison studies attempted to answer the question of whether any such metabolic advantage existed but could not, because not enough dieters completed the study to allow for a statistically valid conclusion.

Another study, which was nicely designed, though smaller and shorter, found no metabolic advantage when it compared a ketogenic low carb diet to a slightly carb-restricted diet that was not ketogenic. In this study, the researchers supplied all the food the subjects ate and the two groups of dieters consumed the exact same amount of calories for five weeks. Half the dieters were fed the nonketogenic low carb diet which contained 150 grams of carbs a day and 50 grams of fat. The other half were fed, on average, 33 grams of carb and 100 grams of fat. The protein intake for the two groups was almost identical, 117 grams for the nonketogenic dieters vs. 125 grams for the ketogenic group, which is more than enough for most ketogenic dieters.

In this study, the *nonketogenic* dieters lost slightly more weight than the dieters eating the ketogenic diet. But this slight difference in weight loss success wasn't statistically significant, and could have easily have been explained by the fact that the non-ketogenic group started out a bit heavier than the ketogenic dieters, or by any of a number of other small, but possibly significant, metabolic differences between the people in the groups. (Johnston, 2006)

Nevertheless, this study did not support the argument that ketogenic diets achieve better weight losses than non-ketogenic diets that provide the same caloric intake. This suggests that when ketogenic diets result in better weight loss, it is either because the ketogenic dieters lose that extra, glycogen-associated weight or because they ate less than did the other dieters because their flatter blood sugars kept them from feeling hungry.

This is good news for low carb dieters because it tells us that most people do *not* need to eat an extremely low carb diet to achieve the best weight loss result. Any diet that flattens blood sugars and controls hunger should make it possible to lose weight by cutting calories.

On the other hand, while there doesn't seem to be any solid evidence that a ketogenic diet outperforms other diets that provide the same number of calories, they may make it possible to eat slightly more food while *maintaining* a significant weight loss. People active in the online low carb community often report that though their weight loss *stalls* when they eat an amount of calories that in theory should pack on some pounds they don't gain weight. That was my own experience over three years of eating a ketogenic diet.

But this claim hasn't been investigated by any formal research, probably because so few of the subjects in the large studies of ketogenic diets remain on ketogenic diets for very long, and even fewer stay on them after completing their weight loss. And even if this is true, its explanation may have less to do with any magic residing in the ketogenic state than with the fact that a diet that strictly limits carbohydrates makes it impossible to eat most of the high calorie junk foods that add more calories to most people's diets than they realize. When you can't eat the donuts, pastry, chips, soda, and fries that make it so easy to pack on weight, you may find it hard to exceed the calorie level that will maintain your weight.

Does Low Carbing Work Because It Lowers Insulin?

Though we saw in the previous chapter that there is no reason to think that the low carb diet increases insulin resistance, we must be skeptical about the claims of low carb enthusiasts who claim that the low carb diet is superior to others because it lowers insulin levels and decreases insulin resistance.

A study by Dr. Westman run at his clinic, funded by money from the Atkins Foundation, attempts to prove this. Unlike many researchers who only report their results in terms of averages, this team published the fasting insulin levels recorded by the individuals they studied, women with PCOS who were eating a ketogenic diet under medical supervision for 24 weeks.

Most of the young women in the study had only mildly elevated fasting insulin levels which did drop to a normal level, but the one individual in the group whose fasting insulin was abnormally high at the study's start—72.7 μIU/ml—though she saw it decrease significantly on the low carb diet, still ended up after 24 weeks with a fasting insulin of 19.5 μIU/ml, which was still more than *twice* as high as the very top of the normal range for fasting insulin. (Mavropolis, 2005)

Another small study of the effects on a group of overweight women of eating a month-long low calorie, very low carb diet run by a team that included Jeff Volek, Dr. Westman's coauthor on the new Atkins diet book, also purports to prove that eating a ketogenic low carb diet for several weeks reduces insulin resistance. However this study concentrated almost entirely on measuring the subjects' cholesterol, which, as you'd expect, improved.

Like Westman, Volek only measured his subjects' fasting insulin, which started out well within the normal range. His subjects' average started out at 6.9 μIU/ml. At the end of their short low carb diet they had slightly lower fasting insulin levels averaging 5.4 μIU/ml. (Volek, 2004) However this is a very minor change with no particular health implications. A truly high fasting insulin of the kind that might cause negative health effects would be in the range we saw in the previous study where that one subject clocked in at 72.7 μIU/ml.

This suggests that if these low carb diets had any impact on insulin resistance, it was probably because they eliminated any secondary insulin resistance they might have experienced as a result of eating high carb meals. However, fasting insulin, the measurement reported in both these studies, is a poor indicator of how insulin resistant people really are. We can only evaluate insulin resistance accurately by observing how well our insulin lowers blood sugar when it rises after a meal.

A major weakness with Volek's study and the large comparison studies we examined earlier that reported that people eating a low carb diet lowered their insulin resistance, is that they estimated insulin resistance by applying a formula, called HOMA (Homeostatic Model Assessment) to their subjects' fasting insulin and glucose readings. Using this formula, the large comparison studies also found that people eating a *high* carb diet also lowered their insulin resistance.

But researchers have found that the HOMA formula gives inaccurate estimates of insulin resistance in people with diabetes, since its estimates don't match actual measurements made by infusing glucose and insulin and monitoring how much insulin it takes to dispose of a known amount of glucose. (Festa, 2008)

This raises the question of whether the HOMA formula, which was developed using data taken from a population of people eating a normal weight maintenance diet and not tested in dieters, produces accurate results when applied to *any* dieters. The calculation is very dependent on the value of fasting glucose, but any diet that limits food significantly will lower fasting glucose. So a drop in the HOMA-calculated measure of insulin resistance in dieters may be telling us more about a subject's food intake than about how effectively a unit of their insulin disposes of a gram of glucose.

A very small but very well-designed study by Mary Gannon carefully measured how its subjects' insulin levels varied after eating. She studied a group of men with what she called "mild" Type 2 diabetes, who were not taking diabetes medications. They were put on a low carb maintenance diet that provided approximately 100 grams a day of carbohydrate for 5 weeks. At the start and end of their diets, their blood was sampled 46 times throughout a day during which they were fed three meals that had been prepared at the lab.

These subjects were significantly insulin resistant, with fasting insulin levels twice normal. Their insulin levels two hours after eating were also more than twice normal. After 5 weeks of eating a very low carb diet these people's diabetic blood sugars improved dramatically. Their post-meal blood sugar peaks had been peaking at an average of 270 mg/dl at all meals before they started their low carb diets. After the diet, they were peaking at 140 mg/dl after breakfast and dinner and at 155 mg/dl after lunch. This decrease would have been enough to make a dramatic improvement in their health.

But after their diets, their average fasting insulin was *still* almost twice the normal level and their insulin 2 hours after their meals, though it was considerably lower than it had been when they were eating high carbohydrate meals, was still twice as high as normal people's insulin levels. And after their diets, the speed at which their blood sugar dropped and the pattern in which their insulin was secreted were also still highly abnormal. Most importantly, their fasting insulin levels, when measured through the night, were almost identical to what they had been before the beginning of their diets. (Gannon, 2004)

Another short study of 10 men with Type 2 diabetes who were taking oral diabetes medications and were put on a strict ketogenic diet for 2 weeks also published graphs showing their glucose and insulin levels. It documented that after their diets these men's blood sugar became completely normal throughout the day except for their fasting readings taken after waking, which were still in the prediabetic range. Their fasting levels before meals, later in the day, had also dropped to completely normal levels.

But their insulin levels throughout the day, though they were far lower than they had been when they were eating a high carb diet, still continued to be roughly twice normal, just as was the case in the Gannon study. And, just like the subjects in the Gannon study, these men's fasting insulin levels remained very similar to what they'd been before starting their low carb diets. (Boden, 2005)

The fact that the abnormally high insulin levels in these insulin resistant subjects remain far higher than normal after eating a low carb diet reinforces the idea that the only kind of insulin resistance that is corrected by low carb diets, including ketogenic diets, is the secondary insulin resistance caused by exposure to high blood sugars.

Primary insulin resistance, which people appear to be born with, does not appear to be significantly affected by diet, since these insulin resistant dieters continue to have insulin levels twice as high as normal. This raises the question of whether the subject's ability to lose weight on a low carb diet had anything to do with any lowering of their insulin levels, which remained twice as high as normal, and suggests very strongly that it was their lowered *blood sugar* levels that made the difference, instead.

Proponents of the insulin theory may argue that these studies were all short in duration and that it's possible that years of eating a very low carb diet might normalize abnormal insulin resistance. But this doesn't mesh with the experience of those in the online diabetes community who have been eating very low carb diets for five years or more. I have several personal friends with diabetes who have been eating ketogenic diets for longer than a decade and maintaining normal blood sugars the whole time. Even so, if they inject insulin, they still have to inject doses ten times as high as those used by people with diabetes who are insulin sensitive.

This shouldn't surprise anyone who is familiar with research into insulin resistance performed by scientists unconnected with the diet community. Their research suggests very strongly that severe insulin resistance is genetic in origin. For example, one study documented that the young, thin relatives of people who have Type 2 diabetes turn out to be far more insulin resistant than normal people when their insulin sensitivity is measured using a glucose tolerance test. (Straczkowski, 2003)

This finding flies in the face of claims that obesity *causes* insulin resistance. It suggests, instead, that many people who are obese and insulin resistant may have started out *thin and insulin resistant* and that they become obese as they age because the abnormal blood sugars caused by this inborn insulin resistance ramps up their hunger and leads them to overeat.

One way that a genetic defect could cause insulin resistance became clear when researchers found that some obese people, "carry mitochondrial proteins and genes that work abnormally and that these anomalies contribute to generating insulin resistance and a reduced response to physical exercise." (Diabetes in Control: Alterations and Petersen, 2004)

The mitochondrial defects these researchers have uncovered cause insulin resistance because they prevent the normal, efficient burning of glucose. This in turn, causes the glucose they can't burn to be stored in their liver and muscle cells as fat.

Obviously, a person who can't burn glucose properly will do a lot better on a diet that doesn't require them to burn glucose, and this is one reason why a low carb diet may be the best diet for insulin resistant people whose insulin resistance is caused by this kind of defect.

But it's important to realize that the low carb diet doesn't correct the defect, it merely avoids triggering its action. And it's also worth remembering that the link between insulin resistance and weight gain is far from proven. There are plenty of insulin sensitive people who are obese, and plenty of insulin resistant people with diabetes who keep their blood sugar normal and maintain a normal weight.

A study titled, "Insulin-sensitive obesity," makes it clear that despite the fact that overweight, insulin sensitive people may have insulin levels are only 1/3 of those found in overweight, insulin resistant people, and may have body fat that is deposited in different patterns, they still cope with enormous weight problems. You can see this clearly in the photographs of two extremely overweight people, one insulin resistant and one insulin sensitive, that you will find in the study titled, "Insulin-sensitive obesity." (Klöting, 2010)

Will Cutting Carbs Prevent Diabetes?

Many people diagnosed with insulin resistance or prediabetes fear that eating carbohydrates will make them become diabetic and believe that the only way they can avoid having this happen is to eat a ketogenic diet of the kind described by Dr. Bernstein in his books.

While such people will benefit from cutting back on their carbohydrates and achieving truly normal blood sugars, only a small number of people who are insulin resistant go on to become diabetic. The prevalence of diabetes in the U.S. is roughly 8% and has remained close to that percentage for decades, even though the rate of obesity and diagnoses of insulin resistance have grown dramatically over this period.

The small increase in the incidence of diabetes that has occurred is largely attributable to two factors: the lowering of the diagnostic criteria used to diagnose diabetes, which occurred in 1998, and the fact that improved medical treatment is helping a lot more people live to the advanced ages where diabetes, like all forms of metabolic failure, becomes more common.

The group in which we are told diabetes rates are rising the most alarmingly is children, but most children diagnosed with diabetes have autoimmune diabetes whose causes have nothing to do with carbohydrate intake. Type 2 diabetes in children, though you read about it a lot in the media, is still extremely rare. The NIH gives the incidence of Type 2 diabetes in people under age 20 as being .4 per 100,000 or 4 per 1 million. It is almost certain that these children who do get diagnosed with Type 2 have suffered severe genetic damage in the womb, as many develop their diabetes only a year or two after they have begun to eat food. It typically takes adults, even those with genes that predispose them to diabetes, decades to develop Type 2 diabetes. (NIH: Diabetes)

Though the CDC announced in January of 2011 that it estimated that roughly one third of American adults may be prediabetic, (CDC: Diabetes) the CDC has a very poor track record when it comes to making this kind of announcement. In March of 2004, Dr. Julie Gerberding, the head of the CDC, made the statement to the press that obesity caused 400,000 deaths a year. This was trumpeted throughout the media. But a study published by her own organization, the CDC, on April 20, 2005 in *The Journal of the American Medical Association* made it very clear that she'd made up this impressive figure. The CDC's study found that the number of deaths attributable annually to obesity was actually 25,814. Not 400,000. (An Epidemic of Obesity Myths)

One reason many people believe that a low carb diet will prevent diabetes is because they believe that by not eating carbs they can give their beta cells a rest. The theory that you could avoid diabetes by "resting" the beta cells that produce insulin was very much in vogue among some doctors who championed the low carb diet in the 1990s. They claimed you could avoid "burning out" those beta cells if you didn't make them secrete higher than normal amounts of insulin, since all that secreting was believed to exhaust them and made them more likely to die.

This theory turned out not to be true. The UKPDS study, a large, long-term study of people with Type 2 diabetes, many of whom were taking drugs that forced their pancreases to secrete heroic amounts of insulin, showed that people taking the insulin stimulating drugs did not deteriorate faster than people who didn't take them. And further discoveries explained that these drugs stop working not because they had killed beta cells but for other, reversible, reasons. (BS101: Drugs)

It turns out that your beta cells don't get any more tired secreting insulin than your salivary glands get when they secrete saliva. And whatever the actual prevalence of prediabetes may be, most people whose blood sugars are in the pre-diabetic range *will not* go on to develop full-fledged diabetes. That's because these people become prediabetic because they are highly insulin resistant. But most people who are insulin resistant have the ability to grow new pancreatic beta cells that can secrete enough additional insulin to keep them from becoming fully diabetic.

This was clearly demonstrated by researchers from Mayo Clinic who carefully studied the pancreases of a group of overweight people who had died. Some had died without developing diabetes. Others had been diagnosed as diabetic. The researchers found that the pancreases of insulin resistant people who had died without developing diabetes featured abnormally large concentrations of insulin-producing beta cells. In contrast, in the people with diabetes, half to 80% of their insulin-producing beta cells had died off, often just at the point when they were attempting to reproduce. (Butler, 2003)

It turns out that beta cells don't get overworked, they get murdered. And what kills them is not making too much insulin but *glucose toxicity*. That's a fancy term for sugar poisoning, and a growing body of research has found that beta cells start to die when they experience prolonged exposure to blood sugars over 140 mg/dl. (BS101: Research)

So why don't the unfortunate 8% of Americans who do develop Type 2 diabetes grow more beta cells, too? The answer appears to be that something keeps them from being able to produce enough of these new beta cells to avoid complete pancreatic meltdown.

The explanation for why this might be isn't clear, but it may have something to do with the fact that most people who develop Type 2 diabetes have one of many newly identified diabetes genes. In people of Western European ethnic heritage, these genes include TCF7L2, HNF4-a, PTPN, SHIP2, ENPP1, PPARG, FTO, KCNJ11, NOTCh3, WFS1, CDKAL1, IGF2BP2, SLC30A8, JAZF1, and HHEX.

People of non-European extraction who develop diabetes have different diabetes genes — which is why their diabetes often doesn't behave the same way as that of Western Europeans. Some of these genes are the UCP2 polymorphism found in Pima Indians and the three Calpain-10 gene polymorphisms found associated with diabetes in Mexicans. Research into the impact of diabetes genes has found that the more of them you have, the more likely you are to be diagnosed with diabetes. (BS101: Causes)

Most of these diabetes genes turn out, upon investigation, not to cause insulin resistance, as doctors had expected, but to impair the ability of the pancreas to secrete insulin. So what might be happening is that people with genes that make them secrete less than normal amounts of insulin have a harder time keeping their blood sugars below the level at which glucose toxicity murders beta cells faster than they can grow new ones.

Whatever the explanation, if you keep your blood sugar at truly normal levels—under 120 mg/dl if possible, and, at a minimum, below 140 mg/dl at all times, you should be able to prevent *your* insulin-producing cells from dying of glucose toxicity.

So the takeaway message here is that your chances of developing diabetes have more to do with your genes than your diet, and everything to do with how carefully you avoid prolonged exposure to high blood sugars.

Most insulin resistant people who don't have diabetic relatives will not progress to diabetes no matter what diet they eat. Those who do, the people who have inherited diabetes genes that keep them from secreting insulin properly, *will* benefit from eating a low carb diet that keeps their blood sugars under 140 mg/dl at all times, since that will prevent glucose toxicity. How many grams of carbs you must eat to keep your blood sugars in the safe zone depends, as we've said earlier, on your own, individual glucose response which can be determined using the technique you'll read about in Chapter 9.

The good news is that even if you do have these unfortunate genes or, for that matter, full-fledged diabetes of any type, you can avoid developing the classic diabetic complications by keeping your blood sugars as close to normal as possible. The genetic flaws that cause diabetes don't cause complications, high blood sugars cause them. And cutting down on how much carbohydrate you eat will greatly improve the blood sugars of anyone with diabetes, a topic that is discussed at great length on my web site http://bloodsugar101.com and on its blog.

Does the Low Carb Diet Lower Thyroid Hormones?

Controversy rages within the online low carb community as to whether eating a ketogenic low carb diet depresses thyroid function. There is some research that suggests it does, and that it does so in a manner that won't be detected by the tests most doctors order to evaluate thyroid function.

This research, almost all of it conducted in the 1970s and 1980s, found that ketogenic diets lowered the levels of T3, the active form of thyroid hormone while they increased the level of reverse T3 (rT3), a largely inactive form of T3 that does not produce the effects on the body that regular T3 does. When most doctors test for thyroid abnormalities they test for TSH, and even the tests that measure T3 may not distinguish between the active and inactive forms.

Unfortunately, there are major problems in interpreting how relevant this research is to low carb dieters. The diets used in this research were either very low calorie diets, of less than 800 calories a day, which will slow the thyroid no matter what the mix of nutrients might be, or they were so low in protein that the only way the ketogenic dieter who was eating such a diet could get the glucose their brains needed was by cannibalizing muscle.

These studies were also very short—lasting only a few days to a few weeks—and did not give the ketogenic dieters time to adapt to their new diets. Lastly, these diet studies fed subjects lab-created liquid diets, many rich in corn oil. None examined people who had been eating real world diets made up of normal foods for any significant period of time. (Paleohacks:T3)

So, for now, we don't have reliable research data that could tell us if eating ketogenic diets that supply sufficient protein would have this same impact on thyroid hormones. Nevertheless, anecdotal reports do suggest that some people who eat ketogenic diets for more than a few months do experience symptoms that suggest lowered T3. These symptoms include failure to lose weight even when calorie levels are low enough that weight loss should occur, exhaustion, hair loss, and lowered body temperature.

Years ago, Dr. Eades posted on his web site that he sometimes prescribed supplemental T3 (cytomel) for some of his patients on long-term low carb diets for this very reason.[14] In addition, since no research examines what happens to T3 in people who have abnormal blood sugars or who start out with marginally functioning thyroids, we have no data to tell us whether the risk of thyroid slowing rises in these special populations when they eat a very low carbohydrate diet.

---

[14] A person posting on Dr. Bernstein's online bulletin board reported that when contacted, Dr. Eades denied having written this, but I was able to find an archived copy of his 1990s web site on the Wayback Machine web site that contained his account of doing this with some patients. I have also heard from a patient of Dr. Richard K. Bernstein's who had been eating a diet of 30 grams of carbohydrate a day who had been prescribed T3 for this kind of lowered thyroid function.

What research we have suggests that when people aren't eating starvation diets, any thyroid slowing due to carb restriction fades out when the carbohydrate intake rises over 105 grams a day. (Pasquali, 1982)

This is, perhaps not-so-coincidentally, the carbohydrate intake level at which quite a few people who have maintained a significant weight loss achieved on a low carb diet report they feel best while they maintain. That's been true for me, too.

Because it takes a while to reverse any changes in thyroid hormone function caused by T3 turning into reverse T3, it may take a while before you see an improvement in your energy level after you raise your carbohydrate intake. Testing for the T3/rT3 ratio is not mainstream, nor is supplementing with T3. However you can find a list of doctors who are open to exploring this kind of treatment at thyroid disease patient advocate Mary Shomon's web site's "Top Doctors" page:

`http://www.thyroid-info.com/topdrs/index.htm.`

Does Eating Carbs Cause Insulin Resistance?

Though we have just learned that some insulin resistance is caused by genetic errors and that lowering our carbohydrate intake does not appear to improve primary insulin resistance, the authors of many low carb diet books tell us that the main reason most of us are insulin resistant is because we have been eating diets high in carbohydrates. From this it follows that the only way to prevent insulin resistance is to cut almost all the carbs out of our diets.

Though there is no doubt that cutting back on carbohydrates will normalize the elevated blood sugars caused by insulin resistance, there is no evidence that people with normal insulin resistance develop insulin resistance as a result of eating carbs. We noted in Chapter 2 that the blood sugars of normal men consuming a meal of almost 500 grams of carbs did not rise out of the completely normal range. By the same token, I and other people with diabetes who have measured our relatives' blood sugars after meals have found that some of them can consume an entire Thanksgiving feast, complete with several slices of pie, and register blood sugars under 100 mg/dl 90 minutes later.

Normal people can eat diets rich in carbohydrates throughout their lives without developing insulin resistance, even though, as we just explained, they may grow quite fat. What a growing body of research has made crystal clear, is that it isn't people's food choices that are making them insulin resistant but the toxic impact of a whole host of organic compounds, most of them not known to nature, that saturate our environment, thanks to industrial practices that have become widespread over the past 50 years.

These chemicals, which can be detected in many people's blood-streams in measurable quantities, have damaged people's bodies in ways that make them far from normal, and disrupt the complex feed-back loops, made up of hormones, that keep normal people from over-eating or experiencing high blood sugars. Once our bodies have been damaged by these chemicals, they can't process carbohydrates the way a normal person's can, and, after that damage has been done, eating carbohydrates will cause significant problems.

Pervasive Organic Toxins Cause Insulin Resistance

Though as we noted earlier, some people are born with defective genes that make them insulin resistant when they are young and slim, you don't have to be born with damaged genes to end up with mito-chondria that can't burn glucose properly. The water you drink may carry a potent herbicide that will damage your genes the same way.

The title of the study that discovered this is, "Chronic Exposure to the Herbicide, Atrazine (ATZ), Causes Mitochondrial Dysfunction and Insulin Resistance." It explains "There is an apparent overlap between areas in the USA where the herbicide, Atrazine, is heavily used and obesity-prevalence maps of people with a BMI over 30. (Lim, 2009)

This study points out, "One such pathway by which ATZ or its me-tabolites might be introduced into humans is through corn-derived foods (e.g., high fructose corn syrup or corn oil)." It continues, "Re-cently, it was reported that of 160 food products purchased at a fast food restaurant throughout the USA, not a single item could be traced back to a non-corn source." It concludes by explaining that atrazine concentrations are highest in groundwater in regions in the United States where corn is processed by soaking it in large amounts of wa-ter—a process called wet milling.

Another class of toxic organic compounds that have been repeatedly linked to the development of diabetes and obesity are the organochlo-rines. They include PVC plastics, PCBs, solvents, and a large number of pesticides including DDT, dicofol, heptachlor, endosulfan, chlor-dane, aldrin, dieldrin, endrin, mirex, and pentachlorophenol.

For example, a study titled, "Diabetes in Relation to Serum Levels of Polychlorinated Biphenyls and Chlorinated Pesticides in Adult Native Americans" found that people who had the highest levels of PCBs in their bloodstreams were four times as likely to be diagnosed with di-abetes as those with the lowest. People with pesticides and fungicides in their blood had an even higher risk. (Codru, 2007) Another study found that the incidence of obesity in toddlers correlated strongly to their mothers' exposure to PCBs. (Mead, 2009)

Insight into how these chemicals make us fat and/or insulin resistant comes from a study of 15 obese people who dieted for 15 weeks. It found that after losing weight, those with the highest levels of organochlorines in their plasma saw their metabolic rates slow the most. As the study report explains,

> The main finding of this study was that the changes in plasma OC [organochlorine] concentration were the main predictor of adaptive thermogenesis, and explained about 50% of its variance. ... this is not a surprise since these compounds produce significant alterations of mitochondrial activity and of the thyroid function. (Tremblay, 2004)

Organochlorines concentrate in animal fat, which is why when you burn fat during a diet, they get released into your blood. They get into your fat in the first place because they are in the dietary fats you consume. For example, a sample of a typical "market basket" of groceries purchased in Sweden in 2005 found significant concentrations of PCBs and toxic flame retardants in fish, dairy products, and, to a lesser extent, in meats. (Törnkvist, 2011)

Though other studies also found pesticides in measurable quantities in commercially sold eggs and meat in other countries, there is a surprising lack of studies investigating the presence of these chemicals in foods sold in the United States. However, what little we have shows that the American food supply does contain measurable amounts of these chemicals, because it is allowable to sell animal feeds that contain trace amounts of pesticides.

Though there are standards for how much pesticide is allowed in our foods, companies whose foods are found to contain dangerous levels of these chemicals are merely given warnings and allowed to continue selling their products, even after repeated violations. And of course, the USDA does not have the resources to test all food sold or all food imported from the many other countries that contribute to our food supply. (USDA: Chemistry)

The food industry and its lobbyists fight all attempts to test for pesticides in the foods shipped to your supermarkets. In addition, they rely on decades old estimates of what constitutes a "safe level" for these toxins—estimates which were never more than a best guess, and which modern research suggests allow us to be exposed to amounts of these chemicals in our foods that go a long way to explaining the so called "obesity epidemic."

Plastics Cause Insulin Resistance, Diabetes, and Obesity

Plastics are another class of organic compounds that interact disastrously with our genes.

BPA

Bisphenol-A (BPA), which is found in the linings of most cans, and, in a finely powdered form, on cash register receipts, has long been suspected of causing obesity. Now we know why. A study published in 2008 reported that, as reported by Science Daily, "BPA suppresses a key hormone, adiponectin, which is responsible for regulating insulin sensitivity in the body and puts people at a substantially higher risk for metabolic syndrome." (Science Daily: Toxic)

As if that weren't bad enough, a research report published in 2011 reported that the level of BPA actually measured in people's bodies after they consumed canned soup turned out to be much higher than expected. People who ate a serving of canned soup every day for five days had BPA levels of 20.8 micrograms per liter of urine, whereas people who instead ate fresh soup had levels of 1.1 micrograms per liter. (Carwile, 2011)

Nevertheless, the FDA caved in to industry pressure in 2012 and refused to regulate BPA claiming that, as usual, more study was needed. (FDA: BPA)

Phthalates

Phthalates are compounds added to plastic to make it flexible. They rub off on our food and are found in our blood and urine. A study of 387 Hispanic and Black, New York City children who were between six and eight years old measured the phthalates in their urine and found that the more phthalates in their urine, the fatter the child was a year later. (Teitelbaum, 2012)

A study of 1,016 Swedes aged 70 years and older found that four phthalate metabolites were detected in the blood serum of almost all the participants. High levels of three of these were associated with the prevalence of diabetes. The researchers explain that one metabolite was mainly related to poor insulin secretion, whereas two others were related to insulin resistance. The researchers didn't check to see whether this relationship held for prediabetes. (Lind, 2012)

Chances are very good that these same omnipresent phthalates are also causing insulin resistance and damaging insulin secretion in people whose ages fall between those of the two groups studied here.

Nonstick Compounds Are Also Toxic

PFOAs are a class of fluorine-containing compounds used for nonstick coatings. They are also sprayed on fabric and carpeting to make them stain resistant. Levels of these chemicals are also detectible in most people's bloodstreams. More than 20 years ago, researchers in a study published in 2012 measured the concentration of PFOAs in the bloodstreams of pregnant women. Years later they examined their children when they had reached the age of 20.

The chilling finding was, "...maternal PFOA concentrations were positively associated with serum insulin and leptin levels, and inversely associated with adiponectin levels in female offspring. Similar associations were observed for males." The more PFOA in the mother's bloodstream, the fatter their daughters were 20 years later and the higher their insulin levels. (Halldorsson, 2012)

What's so scary here is that it took 20 years for this finding to emerge, which should make you realize that many of the other industrial organic compounds floating in your bloodstream—and that of forming fetuses—that you have been assured were safe, aren't. Predictably, the industries that profit from these toxic PFOAs are "working with" the EPA and "studying" the problem. All too often, the politicians who bray the loudest about "protecting the unborn" vote down any regulations that might keep these poisonous industrial products out of fetal bloodstreams. (EPA: PFOA)

Drugs Cause Insulin Resistance and Obesity

Several classes of frequently prescribed prescription medications also cause insulin resistance. Some of them even cause diabetes. Among the worst offenders are statins and many commonly prescribed antidepressants.

Statins

Though I have been warning about this on my web site since 2008, the public only learned that statins increase insulin resistance and raise the risk of diabetes in 2012, right after the patent expired on Lipitor, the most profitable of all the statins. The research I'd blogged about in 2008 found that another statin, Zocor, at all doses "significantly decreased plasma adiponectin levels and insulin sensitivity." (Koh, 2008)

The study that got all the press after Lipitor went off patent was the Women's Health Initiative, which studied 153,840 women for decades. It found that patients who had been prescribed certain types of statins had a 48% higher chance of subsequently being diagnosed with diabetes, compared to their counterparts who were not taking statins. (Culver, 2012)

Doctors in the pay of the drug companies who make these drugs were quoted in the media as saying that this shouldn't be a concern since statins prevented heart attacks, which were the worst side effect of diabetes. Apparently these highly paid experts forgot that statins don't prevent the blindness, amputation, and kidney failure that diabetes also causes.

Antidepressants

Evidence is accumulating that the SSRI antidepressants, including Prozac, Lexapro, Paxil, and Zoloft cause both obesity and diabetes. It had been known for years that people who took these drugs became fat and developed diabetes at a rate higher than that of the general population. But the drug companies who market these highly profitable drugs assured doctors that this happened because people who were going to develop diabetes were more depressive than the population at large, and that therefore the insulin resistance and diabetes seen in the population taking these drugs preceded their use of antidepressants.

This hypothesis was tested in a study published in the journal *Diabetes Care* in 2008. The researchers examined a huge population of people involved in the Diabetes Prevention Program Trial (DPPT). These people did not have diabetes, but had family histories or other factors that suggested they were at risk. They were assigned various interventions including exercise, dietary change, or metformin to see if any of them would prevent them from developing diabetes.

What this study found was that there was a strong link between taking an SSRI antidepressant and developing diabetes, which correlated *not* to being diagnosed with depression, but *only* to taking an antidepressant drug. (Rubin, 2008)

Another, unrelated, study confirmed this finding when it analyzed 10 years' worth of Canadian population data and found that "... the risk of obesity was not elevated in association with MDE [a Major Depressive Episode], ... Unexpectedly, significant effects were seen for serotonin-reuptake-inhibiting antidepressants [Prozac, Celexa, Lovox, Paxil, Zoloft] and venlafaxine [Effexor]. (Patten, 2009)

The class of antidepressants called "atypical antipsychotics" has an even worse track record for causing permanent insulin resistance and diabetes. This class includes Zyprexa and Abilify. A nasty court case in 2007 made public company memos that showed that as early as February 2000, Lilly, the maker of Zyprexa, had found that patients taking

Zyprexa in clinical trials were 3.5 times as likely to develop high blood sugar as those who did not take the drug.

Another Lilly report, from November 1999, showed that the drug company had found, after examining 70 clinical trials, that 16% of patients taking Zyprexa for a year gained more than 66 pounds. (Berenson, 2006)

Some people really do need these drugs and without them would spend their lives institutionalized. For them, the catastrophic side effects may be worth it. But it is well known that SSRIs and atypical antipsychotic drugs have been aggressively marketed to people who are quite capable of functioning without them, and that they are prescribed for conditions they were never meant to treat—including the mild, transient depression that is a normal part of growing up in an imperfect world.

But drug companies have spent billions to convince family doctors untrained in psychiatry to put their patients on these powerful, dangerous drugs at the first sign of depressive symptoms. The many millions of prescriptions they have been writing for these damaging drugs have made huge numbers of people insulin resistant who might otherwise have remained normal.[15]

The conclusion we must draw from data like this is that it isn't carbs that are evil—the real evil is the growing number of substances we are exposed to that damage our ability to metabolize carbs the way human beings have done for millennia. Cutting carbs can keep us from suffering the damage caused by abnormally high blood sugars, but eating carbs isn't causing the epidemic of insulin resistance and obesity.

The best way to prevent future generations from having to turn away from an entire category of human food is to take political action now to limit the ability of unregulated industries to flood our air, water, and food with chemicals that they claim are safe, based only on the manufacturer's own, carefully manipulated research.

---

[15] Tragically, these same SSRI drugs may also be contributing to the surge in the number of children being born with autism spectrum dis-orders. You haven't heard about this research for the same reason you didn't hear about the research linking statins to diabetes. Most SSRIs are still under patent and obscenely profitable. (Croen, 2011)

Points to Remember from This Chapter:

1. There is no conclusive proof that a ketogenic diet allows you to lose weight while eating more calories you do eating other diets, but neither has this been disproven.

2. Low carb diets do not appear to affect primary insulin resistance, though lowering blood sugar will remove the secondary insulin resistance caused by exposure to high blood sugars. It is not likely that low carb diets promote weight loss by lowering insulin. Their effect on lowering blood sugar is the more likely explanation.

3. People with insulin resistance and prediabetes rarely develop full fledged diabetes unless they have diabetes genes that limit their ability to secrete normal amounts of insulin. Diabetes appears to occur after years of exposure to high blood sugars kill off insulin-producing beta cells faster than they can be replaced.

4. It is not clear if ketogenic low carb diets lower levels of active T3. Raising your carbohydrate intake over 105 grams a day should remedy this if it does.

5. Eating carbohydrates is not what causes insulin resistance. Toxic exposures to pervasive organic compounds in the environment probably explain the huge increase in insulin resistance that has occurred over the past 50 years. These toxins include herbicides, pesticides, antistick compounds, PCBs, plastics, and commonly prescribed drugs, including statins and SSRI antidepressants. Keeping your blood sugar normal by cutting carbs will protect you from the damage high blood sugars would otherwise cause. But as long as society ignores this pollution, many people, including children in the womb, will continue to suffer damage that could have been avoided.

Chapter 8
How Much Do Real People Lose?

The peer-reviewed studies we looked at earlier make it sound like weight loss on a low carb diet is modest at best, because they almost always report their results as averages. Dieters who start out weighing, on average, over 200 lbs achieve an average loss of a mere 15 pounds over the course of a year, much of which they regain over the following year. But web discussion forums are full of people who brag they have lost 100 pounds or more on these diets, and the books that promote these diets give the impression these huge weight losses are not unusual.

This makes it hard to get a realistic idea of how effective the low carb diet really is.

On the one hand, we know that some people who post on the web *are* lying about their weight loss. For example, in 2002 a woman showed up on the Lowcarbfriends.com support forum and posted thousands of messages under the name "Kim Kimmer," in which she described an extreme low carb/low fat diet on which she claimed to have lost a lot of weight. She called her diet the "Kimkins diet." Eventually she set up a web site—which is still online —that displayed her before and after pictures and offered visitors an expensive diet plan.

Kimmer's weight loss success was featured in *People* magazine and in the checkout-counter magazine *Woman's World*. Eventually it emerged that Kim Kimmer was actually a 300-pound woman named Heidi Diaz. The post-weight loss photos she had posted turned out to have come from a Russian mail-order bride web site. As a result of investigations that followed a lawsuit brought by people who had signed up for her expensive diet plan, it was revealed that Diaz's web site had taken in $1,200,000 during the month of June, 2007 alone. (Consumer Affairs: Kimkins)

When you realize that an amateur can make that kind of money lying about their diet, you begin to understand the problems we run into when we try to learn the truth about any diet. There's just too much money to be made by selling diet miracles.

But despite the frauds and the many diet book authors who exaggerate their diets' powers there *are* real people getting real results with the low carb diet. I have met several of them in person, both dieters dieting for weight loss and people with diabetes who eat a low carb diet to avoid getting complications. I've also interacted with many more online since I first joined the alt.support.diet.low-carb newsgroup in 1998. These people, who aren't selling anything, freely discuss the difficulties they run into with their diets, not just their successes.

Years ago, through my interactions with a talented group of just this kind of dieter I was able to collect some useful data that, while it isn't peer-reviewed, can answer some of the questions the published research ignores. The most important of those questions is, "How much weight do real people lose on real low carb diets?"

The poll that answers this question uses data that was collected from posts made to the alt.support.diet.low-carb newsgroup back in 2002, back in that more innocent time when the web was not yet dominated by people trying to sell things. Though the newsgroup was not moderated—anyone could post anything they wanted—spam was rare. A core group of people kept the newsgroup's energy high for six or seven years by stopping by a few times each day to post messages, answer questions, share friendship, and provide low carb diet support to a constant stream of people who had just started low carb diets and were full of questions after discovering these diets were tougher to follow than the bestselling books had made them sound.

One of these people was a woman named Carol Ann, who used to post a monthly "Five Pound Challenge," whose goal was to motivate dieters. At the beginning of each month, participants who hoped to lose five pounds over the coming month were invited to post a message describing when they had started their low carb diet, their starting weight for the month, and their weight loss goal.

As the month progressed, these participants would update their weight loss statistics by posting messages to the newsgroup. In 2003, I analyzed five months' worth of the Challenge data that people had posted to the newsgroup, to answer the question of how much weight these real people eating real low carb diets had lost. The results are summarized in the graphs displayed on the next page.

Though many individuals participated in more than one monthly challenge I analyzed the data only on a per month basis, so a person who contributed data to more than one monthly challenge is treated as a separate person in each set of data points.

How Was the Data Analyzed?

I tabulated the 226 individual reports that provided all the necessary data, after breaking them into two groups. Dieters who had been on a low carb diet for less than a month were put into one group, identified as the "newbie" dieters. These were people who were likely to be burning off of their glycogen and losing the associated water weight which I expected would increase their monthly weight loss. Dieters who had been eating a low carb diet for at least a full month were called "experienced dieters" and put into the second group.

The reports were then grouped by the starting weight of the participants at the beginning of the challenge month and by the dieters' gender, where it could be determined from the participant's name. If their gender was not clear from their name, the participant was not included in the gender analysis.

What Did the Data Show?

The graphs below summarize the data, showing the highest, lowest, and median pounds lost for various sub-categories of dieters. To jog your memory in case it's been a while since you've studied statistics, the median is the middle number in a given sequence of numbers. For example, if the pounds lost for each person in a group of nine were 3, 4, 4, 4.5, 4.5, 5, 5, 10, and 14 lb, the median pounds lost would be 4.5 lbs, the 5th value in the series.

In each of the graphs below the dieters are broken into subgroups based on their weight at the start of the month. The number of participants who fell into that weight range is given in the brackets. Each bar shows the median pounds lost and the highest and lowest pounds lost for each subgroup.

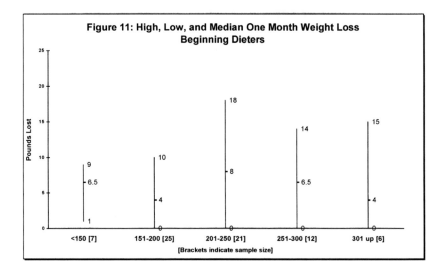

As you can see, there was a wide range of weight losses logged by these beginning dieters, and each group, except for the group that started out weighing 150 lbs or less, included some dieters who lost no weight at all. There were also dieters in each group who lost a lot of weight—9 to 18 lbs. However, though it is not shown these graphs, the median weight loss of the *entire* group of beginning dieters was only 6 lbs, or 1.5 lbs a week.

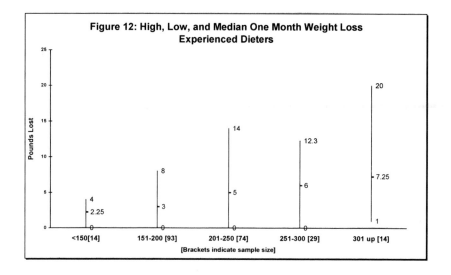

One reason for this relatively low median, in view of how high some people's reported weight loss is, is that not all the beginning dieters made it through the month. The explanation for why some of the newbie dieters lost far more weight than any experienced dieters was, of course, that the newbies who stuck to their diets burned off their stored glycogen and the four times as much water that is stored with that glycogen, as discussed in Chapter 2.

Another factor that can increase the weight loss seen in the early days of a diet is that when people cut way back on how much they eat, they end up with less food in their digestive tracts, so the scale drops by the weight of that uneaten food, too.

When we turn to the data collected from people who had been dieting for more than a month, the median monthly weight loss for all sub-groups of experienced dieters fell between 2.25 and 7.25 lbs. Though it isn't shown on the graphs, the median weight loss for the entire group of experienced dieters was 4 lbs per month, or one pound a week.

It's important to note, though, that in every subgroup analyzed, the median weight loss rose as the starting weight of the dieters increased.

This is so important that I'm going to repeat it in slightly different wording: *The more you weigh, the more you can lose in a month.* This fact has another even more important corollary: *as your weight drops, your rate of weight loss will slow.*

As you can see, in each group there were people who lost no weight over the entire month, except for the group of dieters who started out above 300 lbs. These people who lost no weight were usually people who had been on the diet for longer than 6 months. As you'll recall, many studies show that weight loss slows or stops after that point.

Another reason that weight loss slowed for some of these dieters is that they had lost more than 10% of their starting weight. Once that happens, the hormones that fight to put fat back on your body come into play. So the 201 lb dieter who has dieted down from 250 lbs will find it a lot harder to lose two pounds in a month, while the 201 lb dieter who just started her diet a month before may drop an exciting 14 lbs.

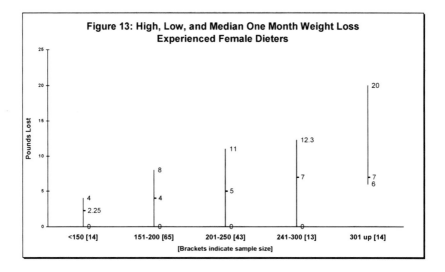

Figure 13: High, Low, and Median One Month Weight Loss Experienced Female Dieters

Gender Differences

Most women, if asked, will say that it seems like men find it a lot easier to lose weight than women do. It is certainly true that some of the most vocal low carb enthusiasts you will encounter online are men who have lost a great deal of weight within a relatively short time. But in this study, the differences between men and women were minor in every group that had significant male/female participation. However, there were significantly more females participating in this study than males.

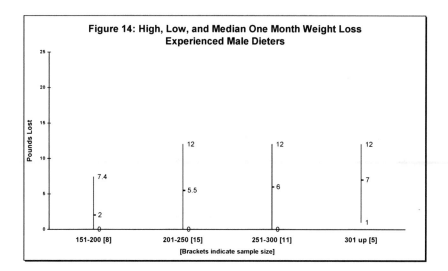

Figure 14: High, Low, and Median One Month Weight Loss Experienced Male Dieters

Points to Remember from This Chapter:

1. A realistic monthly weight goal for a brand new low carb dieter is about 6 lbs, with some dieters losing between 9 and 18 lbs, though most of this weight loss is due to the loss of glycogen.

2. A realistic monthly weight loss goal for the low carb dieter who has been dieting for more than a few weeks would appear to lie between 2 and 6 lbs, with heavier dieters losing a bit more than thinner ones.

3. The longer you've been dieting, the less you should expect to lose each month.

4. Men and women of the same weights appeared to lose at similar rates in this analysis, but we didn't have enough male data to state this categorically.

Chapter 9
How Low Do You Need to Go?

Now that you understand what cutting carbohydrates does to your body, you have the tools you need to craft your own low carb diet. Note that the emphasis here will be on finding your *own* diet. Because no generic diet is likely to work for you over long term, no matter how many degrees the doctor promoting it lists after his name.

My surveys of people who have stuck to their low carb diets for many years make it clear that a major reason why successful low carb dieters *are* successful is because they have found a way of eating that they enjoy—one that not only improves their health but also fits their personalities, philosophical beliefs, and emotional needs. Though they may seem disciplined, they don't succeed because they have abnormal amounts of willpower. Instead, they have found diets that don't require that they exert a lot of willpower because they are comfortable eating them and enjoy the food.

Some of these successful low carb dieters eat stringent Atkins or Bernstein-style ketogenic diets. Other, equally successful, low carb dieters eat 110 grams of carbs each day. Some live mostly on meat. Others eat vegetarian low carb diets where beans provide their major source of protein. Some successful low carb dieters never touch grains, others, equally successful, do. Some count only their carbs, some their calories, and some their visits to the gym or minutes on the treadmill.

These successful low carb dieters have all managed to stick to their diets for at least three years. They have greatly improved their weight and blood sugar control. But what works for any one of them may not work for you, because their genes and metabolisms may be different from yours, and most importantly, so might be the way their blood sugar behaves.

This is why the bestselling diet books can only take you so far. Each book's message tends to be, "This way is the only way." And though there are many people for whom the diets described in these books may work very well, there are just as many for whom they fail.

The diet that will work for a basically healthy though overweight 31 year old male can be very different from the one that works for a menopausal woman with diabetes or a 30-something ex-vegan who has developed gluten intolerance from eating too much soy. By the same token, the diet that works brilliantly for a homemaker who cooks all her meals from scratch in her own kitchen may be impossible to follow for a salesman who spends his life in airports and hotels and must lunch daily with clients.

There is really only one diet-related factor that is, essentially, non-negotiable: Whatever diet you choose must keep your blood sugar in the range that does not raise your risk of having a heart attack or cause the other problems blood sugars do when they spend a lot of time above the truly normal range.

How tightly you want to control your blood sugar is up to you. Those of us with diabetes may have to struggle to get our blood sugars anywhere near normal and may do better shooting for a blood sugar target that is a bit higher. Keeping our blood sugars under 140 mg/dl at all times, to the extent that is possible, will prevent all the classic diabetic complications and greatly reduce our risk of heart disease, even though this level is slightly higher than true normal.

Keeping your blood sugar under 140 mg/dl at all times will also eliminate any secondary insulin resistance caused by exposure to high blood sugars. This will make it easier both to lose weight and maintain blood sugar control.

People who keep their blood sugars under 140 mg/dl often find that they also lose weight, sometimes quite a bit. But more importantly, people with Type 2 diabetes or severe insulin resistance, by choosing a blood sugar goal that is *good enough*, as opposed to perfect, may make it possible to eat a diet that is not so stringent and restrictive that it becomes impossible to maintain. As so much of the research we examined made clear, few people can stick with very low carb diets for more than a few months, even when those diets do an excellent job of controlling their blood sugars.

Since we have also seen that, over the long run, eating a perfect diet for a short while and then going off it can result in worse health outcomes than eating no diet at all, a not-so-perfect diet we can stick to for decades may be a better choice, especially for people who risk serious health problems if they let their health deteriorate any further.

People with diabetes who take oral drugs or inject insulin can often keep their blood sugars below 140 mg/dl by limiting their carbohydrate intake to a level somewhere between 70 and 110 grams per day. As we have seen that is an intake level that not only is associated with significant weight loss, but with improvements to lipids, blood pressure, and other important metabolic measurements.

Many insulin resistant people and people who have been told their blood sugar is prediabetic will also improve their health when they keep their blood sugars under 140 mg/dl at all times, because that represents a drop from the higher levels most of them have been experiencing.

If you can do it, it's even better to lower your blood sugar to a truly normal level, which means keeping it below 120 mg/dl at all times. Doing that optimizes your chances of controlling hunger, losing a good amount of weight, and making substantial improvements to your health over long term.

But as ideal as perfectly normal blood sugars might be, our real goal here is not perfection. It's finding a diet we can stick to, unlike all those people in the diet studies. We don't want a diet that makes the pounds melt off like magic for a few months but leaves us feeling deprived and ready to use any excuse to crash off that diet. Our goal is to craft a healthy diet that will leave us slimmer in 5 years than we are now, without our having regained a significant amount of weight in the meantime.

Adopting a less stringent diet may mean settling for weight loss that is better than average though less than ideal, just as it might mean settling for "good enough" blood sugars rather than perfect ones. But a less stringent diet may be the only diet many of us can stick to forever—after the scale stops dropping, after that early 5 month burst of weight loss is over, and after we realize that, just as the song says, forever is a long, long time.

But before you can figure out what diet will be "good enough" for you, you'll have to figure out exactly how your blood sugar is performing, because a more relaxed diet that continually pushes your blood sugar up over that 140 mg/dl level is not healthy. It will make you hungry and derail your ability both to lose weight and to maintain it. Over time it will also make you more likely to develop heart disease, no matter how much weight you lose.

Fortunately, the wide availability of home glucose meters makes it easy to assess how your blood sugar is behaving and figure out exactly how much carbohydrate it would be healthy for you to eat.

What You'll Need to Test Your Blood Sugar at Home

In order to test your blood sugar at home you'll need a blood sugar meter and a container of at least 25 test strips. In most places you don't need a prescription to buy the meter or strips. You can also borrow a friend or family member's meter. But if you do that, buy your own strips. Strips are expensive, and old ones that have been open for some time may give inaccurate readings.

If you borrow a meter, you will need a brand new lancet needle. The lancet is the device that holds the needle used to poke your finger and get the tiny drop of blood you test. Never use anyone else's lancet needle, as doing so can transmit hepatitis or AIDS. You can borrow the device that holds the lancet needle, but you must *always* use your own lancet needle and never share it with anyone else. It's fine to reuse the same lancet needle for your own use for as long as a couple months. Some people find they are more comfortable after they've been broken in.

If you can't borrow a meter, you can buy an inexpensive meter and strips at a drug store or Wal-Mart. The Walmart Relion meters and the house brand drugstore meters sold at pharmacies like CVS and Walgreens are much less expensive than branded meters and they should come with a lancet device and needles.

Some meters also come with 10 free strips, but not all do. At the store, read the box carefully to see if the meter you have bought includes strips. If it doesn't, buy a box of 25 or 50—whichever is the smallest size available. Strips do not keep for very long once opened, so don't buy more than you need for a couple days worth of tests.

Before you start your test, familiarize yourself with the instructions that come with your meter so that you know how to run a blood test. When drawing blood, don't stab your fingertips. You'll find the fleshy part of the side of your finger next to your nail is much less sensitive. Adjust the lancet device so that it only goes as deep as is needed to get a small drop of blood. Even though the book that comes with your meter says you can, don't test your blood sugar by poking your arm. Not only is this more painful than poking the side of your finger, but the test result is likely to be inaccurate.

Practice a few times before you run your official test. Each meter is different. Be sure you understand how yours works. If you are not in the United States you must convert the blood sugar values given in mg/dl in this book into the mmol/L units used in your country. You do that by multiplying them by 18.

Despite what it says in the instructions that come with new blood sugar meters, it is not necessary to run a test with the control solution that comes with the meter. I have never yet seen a control solution test turn up a problem with a meter, even when my meters had serious problems with accuracy. Running control solution tests just wastes expensive test strips.

Your Meter's Margin of Error

Your meter's result is not as accurate as a lab-drawn test would be.

When I have taken three different meters to the lab with me and tested my blood sugar within a minute of a lab draw, the meter readings at times have varied dramatically from the value reported by the lab. Once, when the lab reported that my fasting blood sugar was 99 mg/dl, my Ultra Mini read 103, my Freestyle Lite read 92, and a Relion Micro read 126.

This may not be entirely the meters' fault. I have been told by someone whose lab-drawn blood sample was sent to two different labs by mistake that the labs returned two different blood sugar readings from the same sample. Measuring blood sugar is, apparently, tougher than we'd like it to be.

Even so, the results you will get from testing are close enough that you can use them to determine how close your blood sugar is to normal. Thousands of people use them to normalize their blood sugars and the results they get when they go to the lab for testing verify that the strategy works.

If you do see a disturbingly high value when you run your home test, don't panic and decide you are on your way to diabetes. Wash your hands and test again. Traces of food on your fingers can cause very high readings.

If you keep seeing readings that are over 140 mg/dl when you test after meals, your blood sugar may, in fact, be higher than desirable. To rule out the possibility that your meter is reading high, try a different brand of meter and see if the results change. If your readings are consistently over 180 mg/dl they are definitely abnormal, even if there is some meter error.

If you see an unexpectedly *low* value—especially any reading under 70 mg/dl fasting—it is possible you haven't let the test strip absorb enough blood, though with the newer meters this is no longer the problem it used to be.

Fortunately, even with this variation, your home meter is accurate enough to allow you to figure out exactly how much carbohydrate your body can tolerate.

Performing the Meal Test

The way you determine how your blood sugar is performing is to eat a normal meal and test your blood sugar one and two hours after you eat it. Some research suggests that this is a much better way to assess blood sugar than the glucose tolerance test that conscientious doctors traditionally employ.

For example, a recent study found that testing women with PCOS for insulin resistance using a muffin rather than the glucose tolerance test turned up *more* subjects with abnormal blood sugar patterns than did the glucose tolerance test. (Freeman, 2010)

If you are currently eating a ketogenic low carb diet you can do these tests with your low carb meals, but your test results won't tell you if your overall blood sugar control is truly normal since eating a meal that contains only 6 to 12 grams of carbohydrates often will make even diabetic blood sugars fall into the totally normal range.

People eating ketogenic diets or very low carb diets who don't want to raise their carbohydrate intake for the sake of testing their blood sugar performance can determine how much additional carbohydrate they can tolerate by testing their usual low carb meals in Step 1 below, and then immediately going to Step 3.

How to Test Your Blood Sugar

Step 1: Eat Whatever You've Been Eating and Write It All Down

Eat three normal meals containing the amount of carbohydrate you eat when you aren't on a low carb diet. Do not eat pizza or pasta for this test as they digest slowly and produce blood sugar peaks at unpredictable times.

When to Test:

At each meal, use your blood sugar meter to test yourself at the following times:

Before you eat

1 hour after your meal

2 hours after your meal

Keep a log, and write down what you ate at each meal and what your blood sugar results were. Make a note any time you feel increased hunger during the test.

What you will discover by this is how long after a meal your highest reading comes and how fast you return to normal.[16]

Interpreting Your Reading

The table below shows you a selection of blood sugar readings and their implications. Normal and High Normal are defined using the values reported the Continuous Glucose Monitor Study referred to in Chapter 1.

If your readings after eating a substantial amount of carbohydrate match the definition of true normal, there is no pressing reason why you must eat a very low carb diet. You should be able to lose weight

---

[16] Most people's blood sugar will peak 1 hour after the end of their meal. But if you eat very slowly, test 75 minutes after you ate your first substantial amount of food and do the second test an hour after that test.

on any diet that lowers your caloric intake, be it low carb, low fat, or a low calorie, portion-controlled, mixed diet.

Step 2: For the Next Few Days Cut Back on Your Carbohydrates

If your blood sugars were not normal in Step 1, eliminate breads, cereals, rice, beans, any wheat products, potato, corn, fruit, and sugary desserts. Get all your carbohydrates from veggies. Test your modified meals using the same schedule above. Cutting out carbs in this way will show you what impact you can make on your blood sugar by cutting carbs from your meals.

	Morning Fasting Blood Sugar	Before Lunch or Dinner	1 Hour After Eating	2 Hours After Eating
True Normal	70-91	80s	Under 120	Under 100
High Normal	92-99	90s	Up to 160	Under 100
Heart Safe	70-99	Under 120	Under 140	Under 120
ADA Normal	70-99	not defined	Under 200	Under 140
ADA Prediabetes	100-125	not defined	Under 200	Over 140 Under 200
ADA Diabetes	Over 125	not defined	Over 200	Over 200

In the chart above, ADA stands for "American Diabetes Association." This is the organization that determines what blood sugar levels doctors are told to use for diagnosing blood sugar disorders. The values it defines are the only ones your doctor will consider important. If you value your health, you'll want to stay within the "Heart Healthy" level that prevents blood sugars from damaging your organs, as the ADA diagnostic levels were intentionally set higher than the level at which diabetic complications start to occur.[17]

Step 3: Find the Top of the Safe Range for Carbohydrate Intake

If cutting the carbs out of your meals has given you normal blood sugars 1 and 2 hours after your meals, you can start cautiously adding back small portions of carbohydrates, making sure to test your blood sugar after each meal. Stop adding carbohydrates as soon as you get near your blood sugar targets. If a certain food pushes you over your

---

[17] The ADA is a self-appointed organization, funded largely by drug and junk food companies that has appropriated to itself the right of defining how diabetes and prediabetes should be defined though the levels they prescribe for diagnosis have been proven by a large body of research to be dangerously high. (BS101: Misdiagnosis)

target, but you really want to keep eating it, try cutting back on its portion size until you find a portion size that keeps your blood sugar within range.

Once you have found a few meals that keep your blood sugar solidly in the normal range, use nutritional software to compute how many grams of carbohydrates those meals contain. Be very careful to match the portion size you actually ate to the portion sizes given in the software.

Once you have determined how many grams of carbohydrates these meals contained, you can eat other meals that contain the same amount or less carbohydrate, knowing they will also keep your blood sugar normal, without having to test your blood sugar after eating each one.

Step 4: Use Your Meter to Check and Tweak Your Diet

Use your blood sugar meter any time you have a question about whether a food is appropriate for your diet. Check foods that give you cravings to see if they are causing blood sugar spikes. No matter what anyone tells you, if a food raises your blood sugar over the targets you are aiming for, that food should not be part of your food plan.

Your Meter Can Take the Mystery out of Restaurant Food

Portion sizes pose a threat to the best-intentioned low carb dieter. Few of us can accurately estimate how much food is on our plate, and the problem is particularly acute when you dine out. Restaurant food often hides carbs in places you'd never expect to find them. There can be flour in taco filling or omelets, unexpectedly high amounts of starch in cream sauces and soups, and five times as much food in a "serving" than is in the serving size you find listed in nutritional software.

If your blood sugar rises out of the completely normal range when you eat anything but a low or lower carb diet, testing your favorite restaurant meals with your meter will tell you if they contain more carbohydrate than your body can handle and are raising your blood sugar out of the normal zone.

If Your Home Blood Sugar Test Results Are High

If, after testing, you see several blood sugars higher than 200 mg/dl, it's possible you may actually have diabetes. A low carb diet will go a long way toward controlling your blood sugars. But if your meter tests suggest you are diabetic, you should visit a doctor to confirm the diagnosis. That's because, if you are one of the hundreds of thousands of people whose diabetes has gone undetected for years, you may already have developed some early diabetic complications, including nerve damage or early changes to your retinas and kidneys that need to be screened for and treated.

If you have health insurance and are given a diabetes diagnosis, many insurers will pay for a monthly supply of blood sugar test strips which you can use to fine tune your diet. They will also pay for a more expensive, slightly more accurate meter.

If you discover you have diabetes, you may also benefit from starting certain medications early rather than late. It is a common mistake to think that controlling blood sugar with diet alone, or with herbs and supplements, is healthier than using pharmaceutical drugs. Solid research has established that starting the safe diabetes drugs, metformin and/or insulin, immediately after diagnosis can make big difference in your health years from now. Both work very well when used in conjunction with a low carb diet.

By the same token, if you consistently see blood sugars over 140 mg/dl two hours after you eat high carbohydrate meals, you are probably pre-diabetic and should visit a doctor once a year to get your kidneys and retinas checked, since these diabetic complications actually start to occur when blood sugars are only in the so-called prediabetic range.

If you have either prediabetes or diabetes you can learn more about how to manage it at my web site at http://bloodsugar101.com and by reading the book based on the web site, Blood *Sugar 101: What They Don't Tell You About Diabetes.*

Points to Remember from This Chapter:

1. The key to success is finding a diet that meshes with your tastes, lifestyle, and physiological needs.

2. A good enough diet beats a perfect diet if it makes it possible for you to stick to your diet for five years or more without ever crashing off it.

3. Testing your blood sugar at home with a meter will tell you how many grams of carbohydrate you can eat without raising your blood sugar to the levels that cause hunger and damage your health.

4. Your meter can also help you determine if specific foods, especially those found in restaurant meals, are compatible with your diet.

Chapter 10
Pick a Diet, Any Diet

Now that you've figured out how much carbohydrate your body can tolerate, you are ready to start or tweak your own low carbohydrate diet.

There are two ways you can do this. One is to eat the foods your blood sugar meter tells you are safe. The other is to pick one of the many low carb diets promoted by bestselling books and do it exactly the way the book describes for long enough to test it out. Then tweak that diet to better fit your needs.

Eating to Your Meter

If you have used a blood sugar meter to determine how many grams of carbohydrate you can eat without pushing your blood sugars out of the truly normal range, you can craft a customized, healthy low carb diet by keeping your carbohydrate intake at the level your meter has shown you produces completely normal blood sugars. If you have any doubts about whether you should be eating a particular meal or food, get out your meter and test how it affects your blood sugars one hour and two hours after eating.

Since pasta and some foods high in fat may digest more slowly, if you see a suspiciously low value after eating a meal that contains an amount of carbohydrate you'd expect to raise your blood sugar, test that meal again a few hours later, to make certain it isn't creating a delayed spike.

To use this technique effectively you *must* get a book, software, or a smart phone app that tells you exactly how much carbohydrate there is in a given sized portion of food and look up the carbohydrate content of all the foods you usually eat. A food scale will also be very helpful, because carbohydrate counts are meaningless unless you know how much of any food you are actually eating. A food that is listed as having 10 grams of carbohydrate in your nutritional guide based on a 2 oz serving size will contain 40 grams of carbohydrate if the serving on your plate weighs 8 oz. This happens far more frequently than people realize and is a major reason why people end up concluding that low carb diets don't work.

This technique is especially helpful for people whose blood sugar levels were significantly above normal—those that went into the range over 160 mg/dl after eating a high carbohydrate meal.

If you are dieting to lose weight and take this approach, you will still have to cut down on how much you eat. But controlling your blood sugar should eliminate hunger and make it easier to eat less. I have heard from hundreds of people who have adopted this strategy just to lower their blood sugar, who have been pleasantly surprised to discover that their weight dropped, too, as soon as they switched to eating meals that kept their blood sugar normal, without their having to consciously count calories. This was because their normal blood sugars controlled their appetite.

But losing weight *always* requires that you cut down on your calories, and eating to your meter may not be as helpful for weight loss for people who have blood sugars very close to true normal, since they may be able to eat a lot of high calorie foods without raising their blood sugar. They won't feel hungry, but if they eat when they aren't hungry, just because the food is there, they will definitely not lose weight, and may even gain some.

The value of controlling blood sugars lies in the way it eliminates compulsive, hunger-driven eating. But if you are eating out of habit, not because you are hungry, you will have to pay more attention to what you eat.

Adopt a Tried and Tested Low Carb Diet

If you have trouble limiting habit-driven eating, and do better when given a highly structured food plan, or if you feel safer having some perfect stranger who claims to be a health authority tell you exactly what to eat, you may be happier following a diet laid out in one of the many bestselling low carb diet books.

There are many of them, and new ones come out each year. Each claims that its diet is superior to all others, as well as simpler, more scientific, and more effective. But as we've seen, people lose very similar amounts of weight on all the different low carb diets, and the improvements they make to various health parameters are similar, too.

Read a few books to get an idea of the variety of choices available. Then pick whichever diet seems to fit your tastes in food and the requirements of your lifestyle the best.

Here are some low carb diets that are tested, safe and, based on the experiences of people who have maintained low carb weight losses for long periods of time, effective.

1. The Atkins Diet as explained in the 1992 book, *Dr. Atkins' New Diet Revolution* or as revised by Jeff Volek, Stephen D. Phinney and Dr. Eric C. Westman in *The New Atkins for a New You*. The diet described in Dr. Atkins' 1992 book is one many people in the online diet community prefer. It's the classic ketogenic Atkins diet and it works, though some of the research Dr. Atkins cited to back up his claims about the diet's metabolic advantage and the efficacy of a fat fast has been discredited or disproved. Because this is a ketogenic diet, be prepared to experience a very quick initial weight loss that will come back as soon as you eat a high carbohydrate meal that refills your glycogen. The fat loss this diet causes is slower but real, and the fat you lose doesn't come back quickly.

2. Protein Power. The diet described in the 1999 paperback is very well explained and gives many helpful suggestions about what to eat both at home and in restaurants. It was the diet I followed for years. It's also a ketogenic diet, but slightly less draconian than classic Atkins. Since publishing this bestseller, the authors have written many other books which are more faddish and less informative.

3. The South Beach Diet. The principles explained in this book work well for people with near normal blood sugars. The diet it describes should put your carbohydrate intake closer to 150 grams a day than 100, which is why its emphasis on controlling your fat intake is appropriate. Because it includes whole grains, it may raise blood sugars too high for some people with higher than normal blood sugars.

Use your meter to test the meals it suggests to make sure they will work for you. The weakness of the original *South Beach Diet* book is that it is vague about what exactly you should eat and how you should adapt the diet after its first few weeks.

4. The Paleo Diet. This diet works very well for many people. Some claims made by some paleo diet enthusiasts that theirs is the original human diet are largely fantasy, unsupported by archeological finds or anthropological studies of people living traditional hunter/gatherer lifestyles, but the diet itself is effective and very healthy. There are several different versions available and all have their avid fans and supporters. Some popular books about this diet are *The Paleo Diet* by Loren Cordain, *Neanderthin,* by Ray Audette, and *The Primal Blueprint* by Mark Sisson.

5. The Carbohydrate Addict's Diet. This diet was very popular in the late 1990s and is described in the book of the same name by the Hellers. It works very well for people who have near normal blood sugars and don't have a history of binging.

There are plenty of other low carb diet books. When you check them out, be careful! Some are useful, some are fad diet books written by opportunists looking to cash in, and some are advertisements by sleazy marketers who sell branded supplements or expensive diet plans. Avoid any low carb diet that requires you to cut your calories down below 1,100 calories a day. That kind of diet may take the weight off, but at the cost of slowing your metabolism in ways that may take years to recover from.

Avoid, too, diets built around the use of any one food or supplement for which miraculous claims are made. That's the hallmark of the classic fad diet and unlikely to lighten anything but your wallet. Ignore the claims of any diet book that promises a quick cure. Even the best diets take many months to improve people's health and years to get rid of large amounts of body fat.

If you're on the fence about a book, check out what other books the author has written. If they've also published books that purport to cure cancer or heal chronic diseases, be particularly wary, as this is a warning sign that the author may be out to make a quick profit, not a difference in people's health.

If a book is written by an M.D. especially one who seems to spend more time in the TV studio than in the clinic, look carefully at his or her credentials. Doctors receive no training in nutrition in medical school. They also learn almost nothing about diabetes or other glandular problems unless they specialize in endocrinology. Quite a few high profile doctors have set themselves up as diet authorities, without having spent the years it takes to acquire more than a superficial knowledge of nutrition. This doesn't keep them from turning their pet theories into books, which can earn them millions, even if the diets they expound are ineffective, unrealistic, or even, for some people, dangerous.

I find it telling that endocrinologists, who spend their careers treating people with difficult weight problems, are the specialists least likely to publish diet books — probably because they know from first-hand experience how complex the topic is and how ineffectual most one-size-fits-all diets are for the people who really need help.

Many authors who put the word "Doctor" in front of their names on their book covers are PhDs, not physicians, and may have received their PhDs in fields like sociology or economics that provided no training in physiology or nutrition. This doesn't mean their books aren't any good. Some of the best health books are written by people who have no medical credentials but have the conditions they write about, who have put in the time and effort it takes to learn about them. But it does mean that you should look carefully at what it is these authors base their advice on.

Pick One, Stick to It, Evaluate and Tweak

Once you've picked a diet, stick to it for two months to see if it works for you. If you pick one of the diets described in a book, do it exactly the way the book tells you to. If you are eating to your meter, eat only foods that keep your blood sugars under your chosen blood sugar target. If you are counting carbs, don't guess at how much carbohydrate is in your food. Use a book, software, or a smartphone app to check on each and every food you eat during the first few months.

If you start adapting and changing your new diet before you give it a chance to work as it was designed to, you are likely to join the many people whose low carb diets aren't effective and, as we've seen in the studies, aren't even low carb.

During the first month of your diet, don't eat any food marketed as "low carb." No bars, shakes, tortillas, cereals, imitation breads or desserts. You can try them later, after you've gotten a good feeling for how your body feels when you are eating a truly low carb diet.

This is particularly true of any foods marketed with the name of a specific diet on the label. As you will read in Chapter 13, the company that bears Dr. Atkins' name has a history of selling foods high in carbohydrates as "low carb" diet foods using deceptive nutritional labels. This is probably true of other diet-branded products.

After you've eaten your diet for two months, stop and analyze how you feel about it. Then make whatever changes are necessary to ensure you'll stay happy eating this diet for years to come.

Here are some questions that can help you identify problem areas:

❖   Is your diet providing the weight loss you hoped for?

❖   Does your diet make you feel good physically?

❖   Are you happy with your food choices?

❖   Does this diet fit your lifestyle or are you finding it hard to stick with due to lifestyle issues?

❖   Are you missing some food to the point where you are obsessing about it?

❖   Are you getting enough micronutrients from fresh, low carb vegetables not pills?

❖   Are you eating more or less junk food than you used to eat?

If your answers suggest you aren't completely happy on your diet, or that your diet is not healthy and sustainable over long term, give some thought to how you could alter it to make it better fit your needs. If you're bored with the food, now is the time to go online looking for low carb recipes. If you're living on hotdogs and pork rinds, clear out the fridge and bring home some low carb vegetables, additive-free meats and unprocessed cheeses instead.

If you need to raise your carb intake level, do it slowly, adding no more than 10 grams a day to your diet each week. If there's some food you really miss, eat a small portion of it once a week. You want to nudge your diet in a direction that makes you more successful, not crash off it.

Learn How to Get Back on Your Diet

That said, if you're lucky, some weeks into your new low carb diet, you will crash off it. The reason this is good is because the single most important thing you will have to learn to make your low carb diet a life-long diet is how to get back on it after a slip.

It's been my observation that the most inflexible dieters, the ones who swear no evil carbs will ever again cross their lips, are the ones who are the most likely to let one day of poor food choices trigger the three month binge that packs on all the weight they lost.

This doesn't have to happen. But the secret to keeping it from happening is to be prepared for the inevitable slip that's waiting in your future. If you understand the physiological changes that can happen when you carb up after a period of carb restriction, you are less likely to panic or become overwhelmed by a raging attack of hunger.

Because you've read this far, you're already way ahead of most low carb dieters. You know, as many low carb dieters do not, that the weight you'll regain overnight after a single high carb meal is not body fat, but merely the glycogen and water you lost during the first few weeks of your diet.

You also know that once your glycogen refills you'll only gain fat if you eat more calories than you burn. So the panic that causes many naive low carb dieters to despair when they regain that glycogen-related weight won't send you into a fit of self-loathing that leads to denial and binging.

You also understand why any sudden increase in your carbohydrate intake is likely to make you hungry, knowing that it will push your blood sugar way up and result in the steep drop in blood sugar that will make your brain scream, "Feed me carbs!"

When you carb up, you'll be aware that because you've cut your carbs down for a while, your body may have downregulated the enzymes needed to burn glucose, and that this may make your blood sugar surge even higher than it did before you started your low carb diet, though this is a temporary phenomenon.

If you don't experience hunger cravings after eating your first high carb meal, you may encounter them when you go back to eating your usual low carb diet. That's because after you eat a high carb meal, your body will assume the next one is going to be high in carbs, too, and secrete enough insulin to cover it.

Since that insulin will be more than you need to cover the small amount of glucose your low carb meal produces, it may push your blood sugar below its baseline value, which will raise the level of hunger-stimulating ghrelin and make you ravenous. But it shouldn't take more than a day for this blood sugar-related hunger to stop, if you continue to limit carbs. If you weren't hungry when eating your low carb diet before you crashed off it, you won't be hungry a day or two after you go back to eating that same low carb diet.

When you do slip up, consider it a learning experience. Note how much water weight you put on and how long it takes to go away when you get back on-plan. Observe the way hunger arises and track how long it lasts. As you become familiar with the process, it will get easier to get back on-plan, because you'll recognize the stages, and know that it will only be a matter or a day or so until you are your usual self. Each time you get back on-plan this way, you'll gain a little more confidence that you are in control, not your hunger, and you'll lose the crippling fear of carbs that hampers so many low carb dieters.

When You Keep on Crashing Off Your Diet

If you repeatedly crash off your diet, or if you are thinking of going back onto a low carb diet after recovering from a catastrophic months-long binge that undid all the benefits you'd gotten from your last diet, as happens to so many erstwhile low carb dieters, don't go back to eating the same diet you ate before and expect a different outcome.

Whatever its supposed benefits, your last diet did not meet the ultimate test of a good diet, which is that you could stick to it through thick and thin without needing to be superhuman. Don't blame yourself for being weak and vow you'll be stronger this time. You won't. And you shouldn't have to be. Instead, take the time to analyze what it was that made it impossible to stick to your last diet and change the way you diet this time, so the same problem doesn't derail you again.

The biggest "secret" of diet success is that the people who stick to diets for years are the people who find ways to diet that don't rely on heroic amounts of willpower. They adapt whatever diet they use until it fits their own way of life, their own food preferences, and if their circumstances change, they adapt their diets to fit those new circumstances. Diets don't fail because we are weak; they fail because they aren't matching up with our metabolic or emotional needs.

The most common problems people identify, when they take a long, hard look at why their diets imploded, is that they got bored with the food, felt overly deprived, got physically drained, developed relentless hunger, or found that the restrictions imposed by their diet limited their social life in ways that made them intolerable.

If that's the case, get yourself some low carb cookbooks and experiment with various recipes until you can find a good selection of foods you enjoy eating. Try making a few day's worth of meals and freezing them, so you have foods you like on hand when you get hungry. Go online and read the discussions you'll find in low carb forums to see how other people solve problems like what to eat for breakfast, or what to bring to work for lunch.

If you can't face eating nothing but meat, eggs, cheese, and greens, try a different kind of low carb diet this time, one that lets you eat a bit more carbs and a bit less fat.

If the problem with your old diet was that a few foods you missed eventually became obsessions, let yourself eat small portions of them now and then in a safe situation where the portion size is limited and you aren't going to put yourself in danger of going overboard.

If you felt physically drained or kept feeling hungry, try raising your carb level to 110 grams a day. Some people don't adapt well to ketogenic diets. If that much carbohydrate raises your blood sugar too high, talk to your doctor about getting some help with your prediabetes. Metformin, which is commonly prescribed for prediabetes, is a very safe drug that often dramatically lowers hunger for people who find themselves hungry while eating low carb diets.

Some people's diets always fail just when they get near the point where they might have to worry about becoming more attractive. This may happen because the reason they originally gained weight is tied up with traumatic experiences they suffered in the past and losing the weight makes them feel they will once again be vulnerable. Other people may unconsciously fear that they may destabilize their marriages if they become more attractive. If this describes you, you will need to find a way to deal with these issues if you are to succeed at weight loss.

Some people turn their diets into arenas where they battle with themselves. They struggle against an unending stream of negative self-talk, which eventually pushes them into self-destructive behavior. If that happens to you, you may need to get some help from a skilled therapist who can help you confront the sources of that negative self-talk and learn how to give yourself the love and support you need so you don't interpret a bad day on the diet as yet more proof that you are a terrible evil person who deserves to be punished for your gluttony.

Advice from Successful Low Carb Dieters

To help you fine-tune your diet, I've summarized what a group of successful low carb dieters told me when I asked them what advice they'd give people starting out on a low carb diet.

This group was made up of a mix of dieters with and without diabetes who had stayed on their diets for at least three years. Several had been on their diets considerably longer than that. Some were dieting only for weight loss, some for blood sugar control, and some for both.

These dieters differed greatly in what they had eaten to *get* to their diet goals. Some had eaten ketogenic diets, several were eating Paleo. Some ate carb-reduced diets with higher carbohydrate intakes. Some were eating to their meters, including several who were eating carb-reduced vegetarian diets that are compatible with Hindu religious beliefs.

However, though the foods and macronutrient ratios these dieters ate differ, when asked what advice they would give people who were just starting out on their own low carb diets, these successful low carb dieters agreed on a surprising number of points.

Here's a summary of what they said, along with a list of warning signs that might mean you're ignoring something important that they've learned.

1. Long-Term Successful Dieters Eat Diets Made Up of the Foods they Enjoy Eating. This is such a simple statement its importance may not at first be evident. But it's the key to sticking to any diet. Over and over successful dieters said things like, "I make sure I am always satisfied. I never want to feel deprived or hungry," and "Don't think about what you *can't* have—think about what you *can* eat and what you *choose* to eat."

One very successful dieter explained, "Make sure you enjoy what you're eating—for me that means finding a variety of traditional recipes that fit, so I don't get bored, and it doesn't feel like 'diet food.'"

Another, who was eating low carb to normalize diabetic blood sugars pointed out, "It's important to focus on what you *can* eat, not just on what you can't eat. Be willing to try new foods and new preparations. And think about things you like that are naturally low carb that you don't always eat." As an example, she explains, "I got through the months immediately after diagnosis by eating large quantities of avocado."

Several of the successful dieters suggested that people new to the diet learn how to cook, so that they can provide themselves with a wider and healthier selection of choices than they will find if they rely on in prepared foods or restaurant offerings.

Typically, too, these successful low carb dieters like eating the core foods that make up a low carb diet: meat, fish, poultry, cheeses, eggs, yogurt, and non-starchy veggies. If you hate this kind of food, no matter how theoretically healthy or effective a low carb diet may be, it isn't going to work for you. In that case, a diet that lets you eat a moderate rather than low carb intake, along with a lower fat intake, and careful portion control, might work better for you.

Some of these successful dieters are maintaining large weight losses by eating diets that allow them to eat small portions of high-quality grains now and then. Some say that they do better eating small amounts of whole grain bread than they do eating additive-heavy low carb bread substitutes that reinforce cravings for breads and pastries.

Warning Sign: You Dream of Eating Forbidden Foods. If you keep dreaming of stuffing yourself with something you've declared completely off limits, chances are very good you are heading for a diet meltdown. It may not happen until some life stress pushes you over the edge, but it's waiting for you, and the more you fight it the worse it will get.

The solution may be to find a way to work a small amount of whatever food you are obsessing about into your diet plan. Often a food becomes the object of an obsession because you've forgotten how it tastes. Eating a small portion of this kind of food, away from home, so you won't be tempted to binge on it, may defuse your obsession. Your first portion may taste ambrosial, but when you eat another small portion again, a week later, you may be surprised how quickly it starts tasting like nothing special.

2. Many Successful Low Carb Dieters Recommend You Do a Week or Two of Ketogenic Dieting To Start With and Go Back to It Later When Bad Habits Sneak Up on You. Eliminating all carbohydrates for a week or two is a good way to make yourself aware of how much carbohydrate you've been eating, and it helps break the many carb-rich snacking habits you've developed.

After you've been on a low carb diet for a while, you may become the victim of "carb creep," like so many of the dieters we read about in the studies, and be eating far more carbohydrate than you realize. A week or two of eating a stringent very low carb diet will make you much more aware of the bad habits you might have fallen into and recharge your diet.

Warning Sign: You Don't Have a Specific Target for Carbs, Calories, or Blood Sugar Level—or if You Had One, You've Strayed Far from It. If your original diet turns out to be too vague, come up with some set guidelines to help you keep on track. What they are is up to you. But setting a limit to carbs, calories, the number of snacks, or how often you dine at restaurants where you tend to overeat can all be helpful.

3. Successful Low Carb Dieters Eat High Quality Food. Despite the very real differences in what they choose to eat, a very strong theme that emerged in my poll was how many successful dieters urged beginners to concentrate on eating real foods and to stay away from the imitations of high carb foods that are marketed to the newbie low carb dieter.

"Stay away from fads!" one successful low carb dieter cautioned. Another said, "Avoid 'low carb' products as much as possible. You'll avoid potential weight loss issues and save a ton of money. Another urged new dieters, "Stay away from 'Frankenfoods.'"

Several reported that over the course of their diet they discovered the advantage of "eating clean." One, who lost 150 lbs, explained, "My diet was a slow transition the entire time I was losing weight ... going from crap frankenfoods with artificial sweeteners, etc. to organic healthy whole food. I took it slow so I could make changes, get used to them, and have them become second nature. Then [I'd] change something else."

If you do feel the need to eat foods similar to your old, high carb standbys, make your own at home using pure ingredients. There are plenty of great low carb recipes online that simulate foods you may have given up, ranging from protein pancakes to surprisingly delicious fauxtatoes and pizza crusts made out of cauliflower. Just go to Google and search on "Low Carb Recipes."

Linda Sue's web site, "Linda's Low Carb Menus & Recipes" is a great place to start. You'll find it at:

`http://www.genaw.com/lowcarb`

You can also find many recipes contributed by members of the old alt.support.diet.low-carb newsgroup at Tina MacDonald's web site, "Recipes from the Wonderful Cooks at alt.support.diet.low-carb" which you'll find at:

`http://www.camacdonald.com/lc/LowCarbohydrateCooking-Recipes.htm`

These completely low carb recipes were developed back in the days before there were commercially available "low carb" products.

Warning sign: Your Low Carb Diet Is Heavy on Low Carb Pancakes, Low Carb Brownies, Low Carb Muffins, Low Carb Meal Replacement Bars and Very Little Meat, Fish, and Vegetables. The classic advice to low carb dieters of all persuasions has long been that when you go to the grocery store you should, "Shop the edges." That means buy dairy, meat, fish, poultry, and vegetables, and leave the stuff in boxes alone. It works.

4. Long-term Dieters Don't Treat Their Diets Like a Religion. It is extremely common to see cult-like behavior develop around a diet, complete with leaders, initiations, sacrifices, and the deep conviction that the dieter is superior to those not eating the diet, who will be punished at some future time when the dieter reaps the rewards of self-denial.

This is most likely to happen when a diet works, which is why low carb diets of all kinds have such fanatic adherents and are so prone to develop cult-like behaviors.

But religions that start out with conversion experiences and threaten others with eternal punishment are also famous for their members' fall into depraved backsliding. Just as there are televangelists caught with hookers, there are more low carb dieters than you might imagine sneaking off to Dunkin' Donuts after posting messages on web discussion boards condemning people whose diets are too lax.

If your goal is a lifetime of weight control and better health, you would do best to disassociate the powerful emotions associated with religious conversion from the question of what you should have for dinner. Flexibility not rigidity is the key to long-term success.

Warning Sign: You Feel Angry When You See Other People Eating Carbs and Console Yourself by Imagining They Will Experience Bad Outcomes. There are plenty of people who would be better off if they ate less carbs, and we all have a desire to help others by sharing what works for us. But if you were really satisfied with your own diet, you wouldn't feel a need to make other people eat it too, and you certainly wouldn't feel anger at people who eat differently—many of whom, you might find if you checked out their situation, are in perfectly reasonable health and doing as well as you are with their weight control and blood sugars.

5. Successful Dieters Focus on Health Not Vanity Goals. Over and over the successful dieters I polled explained that their motivation for losing weight and maintaining their weight loss was a desire for better health, not to fit into a smaller size. As one of these dieters explained, "If you are losing weight to 'look good' at a reunion, you will most likely be one of the 95% who fail, because once the reunion is over, what is your reason to continue?" Another said, "I think like a health nut, not a dieter." And mind you, these answers came from dieters who were *not* dieting to control diabetes.

Warning Sign: You cut out all vegetables from your diet and live on meal replacement bars and vitamin pills because that lets you fit into your skinny jeans. We've already seen that all dieters must contend with a hormone system that wants them to regain any weight they've lost. This makes it essential to provide your body with as wide a range of naturally occurring nutrients as possible, in the form of healthy, additive-free foods and to lose weight at a rate that doesn't convince your body you're starving to death.

6. Successful Dieters Don't Hang Up on Unrealistic Goals. They lose what they can lose without making themselves crazy, declare victory, and move on. A dieter who loses ten pounds and keeps it off for ten years is a much more successful dieter than one who loses 100 lbs but regains 110.

No one can tell you what a realistic weight loss goal for you is until you start trying to lose weight. The people I have polled report losses ranging from 6 lbs (for someone maintaining for blood sugar control) to 190 lbs. In one poll I conducted, I heard from 51 people with diabetes who had been successful at controlling their blood sugar for at least two years. The median weight loss they reported was 50 lbs and the median percentage of starting body weight lost reported was 20%. The range of weight losses in this group mostly fell between 10 and 30% of their starting weight.

Tellingly, a few people reported that they had been able to lose more than 20% of their starting weight, but that they ended up regaining to the 20% point because they found that amount of weight loss easiest to maintain.

This experience was echoed by some of the weight loss dieters I polled who weren't conscious of having blood sugar issues. Some reported they "never got to goal" but that they stopped dieting when further weight loss would require eating at too low a calorie level.

Because it is so much easier to lose weight when you are heavy than when you are closer to a normal weight, selecting a *percentage* of your starting weight as a goal rather than a set number of pounds may be more likely to lead to success.

And if you are an older person who is coping with metabolic dysfunction, be it diabetes, thyroid disease, or an inflammatory condition, or if you have severe arthritis or other conditions that limit mobility, losing even 3% of your starting weight may be an achievement that puts you way ahead of most other people who are battling the same challenges.

Warning Sign: You Have Started Trying Increasingly Faddish Diets Because You Have *Only* Lost 50 Lbs but Want to Lose 100. There's nothing wrong with wanting to stay on your diet and lose more weight. The problems arise when you become so frustrated after losing a respectable amount of weight that you let frustration lead you to do things that may, in long term damage your health. Fad diets, if they achieve weight loss at all, do so in a way that damages your metabolism and makes any weight loss they achieve impossible to maintain. Don't let frustration tempt you into employing strategies like cutting your calories to starvation levels, or prohibiting all but a tiny selection of foods. If weight loss has stopped, savor the accomplishment of getting as far as you have. Many people will never get this far, whatever your original goal might have been.

7. Successful Dieters Plan Ahead to Eliminate the Situations They Know Can Derail Their Diets. As one successful dieter explained, "I make sure I am always prepared no matter where I am to have healthy food choices available, rather than be put in a position where I have to eat whatever crappy food just happens to be available." For some this means carrying a few mozzarella sticks in their purse or pocket when they go shopping. For others, it means not going to dine at places where they know there is nothing safe for them to eat.

My mantra has long been, "If it it's not there, I can't eat it," which means that even though I allow myself to eat small portions of off-plan foods from time to time, I don't bring them home. There's rarely anything in the fridge I shouldn't eat. If there is, the chances are I'll eat it. I don't rely on willpower to stay on my diet. I rely on careful grocery shopping.

If you must eat out, don't be shy about asking the server what's in the food you're about to order, and if the server isn't sure, have them ask the chef. Many restaurants will let you substitute a small salad for a potato side dish when you order an expensive sandwich or dinner entree. If they don't, choose someplace else to dine the next time you go out.

Quite a few of the successful dieters pointed out the dangers of giving in to social pressures. "Learn to ignore friends and relatives who try to convince you that one bite or one serving of something won't kill you," said one, explaining that giving in to that kind of pressure is what has repeatedly pushed her weight back up from goal.

Another added, "I don't care if I 'offend' someone by not eating something they made if it isn't something I would normally eat. My health is more important than someone getting their feelings hurt." Others suggest warning friends before accepting an invitation that there are some foods you can't eat, without going into detail. As long as you don't insist *others* can't eat those foods in front of you — which *is* offensive — true friends and people who understand the ground rules of politeness should be glad to accommodate your needs.

If you must go to some event where you know there will be no food you can eat, eat before you attend or bring your own food along. I have brought more than my share of rotisserie chickens to potlucks where the other guests were vegetarians.

Family members can pose more of a challenge, since unlike friends, often believe they *don't* have to treat you with politeness. Many of us find that it's our relatives who try the hardest to make us give up our diet. Before you assume that they are doing this to be destructive, try to find out their motivation. Sometimes it's because you've developed the dieters' dragon breath that *you* can't smell but other people can. If that's the case, cut back on your protein. There is no reason that a low carb dieter has to smell bad.

Others may have been swayed by what they've heard in the media about how unhealthy the diet is and are trying to derail you out of a misplaced concern for your health. In that case, share with them the information you learned in Chapter 6 that debunks the myths that make some people still think that low carb diets are dangerous.

If, as sometime happens, someone's reason for tempting you to eat things you have decided not to eat *is* destructive, avoid them and if that isn't possible, ignore them.

Warning Sign: You Stick to Your Diet All Week but Blow it Every Weekend. If your life is full of situations that tempt you to eat foods you have decided to avoid, you have several choices. You can avoid the situations where you go out of control—for example, bars where you are tempted to drink enough to lose your inhibitions and forget about your diet. You can bring your own food along, if the problem is that you socialize in situations where there are no foods you can eat. Or you can modify your diet to better fit your lifestyle. For example, you might raise your carb intake slightly, eat less fat, and use a calorie-counting, portion-controlled diet strategy.

Points to Remember from This Chapter:

1. The best diet for you is one that you can stick to without raising your blood sugars to harmful levels after meals.

2. You can diet by using your blood sugar as a guide, or you can choose from any number of published diets.

3. Whatever diet you choose, do it exactly the way it is described in whatever book you choose and stick to it for two months. After that, analyze what isn't working for you and tweak the diet to take care of those issues.

4. Successful dieters don't succeed because they have more will power than others but because they find diets that best suit their personalities and physiological needs.

5. Successful dieters eat real food and stay away from processed fake diet foods.

6. Dieters who don't turn their diets into religions but keep them in perspective and treat them as a good way to improve their health do best over the long term.

7. Successful dieters plan ahead and avoid people and situations that they know might derail their diets.

Chapter 11
Side Effects

There are some common symptoms low carb dieters encounter that aren't always explained in books written by low carb enthusiasts. And though they are listed as "side effects" in the research studies, the studies don't say what to do about them. Most of these side effects have very simple solutions, which we'll examine next.

Constipation

This symptom is very common with all low carb diets, mostly because many people, when they start a low carb diet, make the mistake of eating nothing but very dense foods like meat and cheese, and cut out bulky, fibrous vegetables so they can save their carbohydrate budget for treats and snacks.

That is a serious mistake. No one ever got fat eating big plates of broccoli or kale. Many of the successful low carb dieters I've polled emphasized that it is important to eat a lot of healthy, low carb green vegetables like asparagus, artichokes, broccoli, green beans, kale, collards, deep green lettuces, zucchini, cabbage and brussels sprouts. Fresh berries are low in carbohydrates, too, and provide healthful nutrients and bulk.

Ketogenic diets can be even more binding, because when they flush out glycogen they can be dehydrating. Though some people think they can replace this water by drinking more, the water you drink can't replace the water that is gone from your muscles because the glycogen that held that water is gone. Your digestive system is largely made up of muscle, so it shrinks, too.

Most people find that taking a single teaspoon of a psyllium supplement like Metamucil each day relieves the problem. Examine the label closely as some brands contain sugar. Bran crackers can also help keep things moving, or you can buy bran in bulk in the health food department of your supermarket and add it to foods like yogurt or flax meal cereal. Don't take laxatives as they can make the problem worse over time.

Headache and General Weakness

These symptoms are common on ketogenic diets at the start of the diet when your body is making the shift from burning glucose as its primary fuel to burning fat. Some Atkins dieters describe this combination of symptoms as "induction flu," using the term which Dr. Atkins used to describe the first two week of his diet during which dieters eat only 20 grams of carb a day.

These headaches occur as the brain switches to burning more ketones. They may also be caused because burning more fat requires the cells to upregulate certain enzymes and this takes time. During this interim period when the body is making the switch to burning fat, some cells may end up using an alternate, anaerobic, process to produce energy. Anaerobic respiration produces lactic acid, a substance that causes muscle pain and perhaps headaches.

Another reason you may get a headache on a low carb diet is that you aren't eating enough. Some people respond to the hunger-controlling effects of the low carb diet by eating too little which can also make them feel ill.

You may also feel headachy during the early days of a ketogenic diet when your body is burning through glycogen, because you are urinating more than usual and losing electrolytes. Drinking water with a sprinkle of salt substitute that is half sodium chloride and half potassium chloride may be helpful here.

The headachy feelings induced by going into a ketogenic state should pass within a few days. If they persist more than a week, you may do better on a diet that provides a bit more carbohydrate.

Difficulty Sleeping

Many people report that they find it very difficult to sleep in the early weeks of a ketogenic diet. Others report vivid dreams. These are some other side effects caused by the brain switching to burning ketones. It's a short term effect that should stop within a week or two.

The upside of this symptom is that many people who experience this symptom also find themselves feeling highly energized during the day, though that feeling, too, tends to pass with time as the body adapts.

Bad Breath

It is common to call the bad breath that is notoriously common among people eating ketogenic diets "ketobreath," and many people accept that it is something they need to live with if they are to continue losing weight. That's because they believe that bad breath is inevitable when they are in a state of ketosis and burning fat.

This is a major mistake. The bad breath associated with low carbing is a major reason why the friends and family of low carb dieters start undermining their diets. It can make it intolerable to be confined in a car with the reeking dieter—to say nothing of engaging in more intimate contact. The dieter, meanwhile, smells nothing, even if he breathes into his hand and sniffs, and has no idea he is producing toxic fumes every time he exhales.

The usual advice dieters give each other in online support groups is to drink more water or use breath mints, but neither of these solutions solves the problem. Brushing your teeth won't help either, because this kind of bad breath comes from your lungs, not your mouth.

Ketobreath is Often *Protein* Breath.

Fortunately, it is possible to eat even a ketogenic a low carb diet without giving off toxic fumes. Why? Because what often causes the dragon breath associated with ketogenic dieting is *not* ketones, as most people believe, but eating too much protein.

Diet books frequently promote low carb diets as high protein diets because doctors still don't want to be seen as promoting high *fat* diets. As a result, many low carb dieters eat far more protein than their bodies need. It isn't uncommon to run into low carb dieters who are eating 40 ounces of protein a day.

This may be the right amount for a well-muscled 300 lb football lineman, but it's twice as much as a sedentary 220 lb middle-aged woman needs once she has been on the diet for a few weeks and much of her brain has switched to burning ketones instead of glucose. A smaller, 50-year old woman who weighs only 150 lbs needs only 15 ounces of protein each day once her body has adapted to burning fat. That's all it takes to repair her muscles and synthesize enzymes and hormones.

The reason that excess protein causes stinky breath is this: As we explained earlier, any excess protein we eat gets broken down in the liver and converted into glucose. To convert this protein to glucose, the liver has to first extract all the nitrogen from the amino acids that make up the proteins. That nitrogen then gets turned into ammonia.

That is why, if you are eating too much protein, you will often detect a strong ammonia smell in your urine. In some cases this ammonia might even cause a diaper-rash-like irritation. If your bloodstream is carrying more ammonia and related breakdown products

urea

than your kidneys alone can dispose of, those compounds will be excreted through your breath.

The cure for this dieter's bad breath is simple. Cut down on your protein. If you worry about not eating enough you can use the low carb diet protein calculator you'll find at:

http://www.phlaunt.com/lowcarb/DietMakeupCalc.php[18]

Eat only that much protein for a few days. You should see your bad breath problem clear right up. When you cut down on protein, replace some of the calories you were getting from protein with healthy fats like butter, flax oil, coconut oil, or nuts.

Muscle Cramps

Our body keeps sodium and potassium carefully balanced. But if we lose a lot of fluid quickly, as happens when we are burning through our glycogen stores on a ketogenic diet, our potassium levels can drop. The muscles most likely to cramp are the leg muscles, and you may feel as if you have "restless leg syndrome." There is a simple cure for this—supplementary potassium, but it is one you must *not* use if you are taking certain prescription blood pressure medications.

If you are taking any blood pressure medication, talk to a registered pharmacist who can tell you if the drug you are taking is one of the "potassium sparing" blood pressure medicines that make it dangerous to take added potassium. A pharmacist is more likely to give you an accurate answer to this question than a physician. Every pharmacy should have a registered pharmacist on its staff, so make sure you ask your question to the pharmacist, not a pharmacy clerk.

If you aren't taking a medication that could cause a problem, or if your pharmacist gives you the OK to use potassium, the easiest way to supplement with potassium is to use a single sprinkle of a potassium chloride salt substitute. Potassium pills contain such a low dose of potassium that you will have to take a lot of them to see any effect.

If you find a salt substitute that is 100% potassium chloride, use it with care. The reason the doses are kept low in potassium supple-

---

[18] Be aware that if you are severely overweight the calculator may overestimate your protein needs as it uses a formula based on total body weight that doesn't work properly for people whose lean body mass is significantly less than normal. Protein is used mainly to repair and maintain muscle, so if your body is carrying a very high percentage of body fat, the number the calculator will provide may be higher than what you really need. In that case, you would do better to estimate your need by using a formula based on lean body mass and adding to its estimate however many more grams of protein you will need to top up the supply of glucose your brain needs. Remember that 58% of the protein grams you eat can turn into glucose and that an ounce of high protein food like meat, eggs, or cheese, contains 6 grams of protein.

ments is that taking too much potassium can destabilize your heart-beat. A single small sprinkle of salt substitute should be all you need and should alleviate cramps within a few minutes.

Shakiness or Hypoglycemia

Quite a few people report feeling shaky or experiencing what they describe as hypoglycemic attacks when they start a low carb diet. Some find that, when this happens, they become very hungry.

It is normal to experience hypoglycemia after you sharply decrease your carbohydrate intake. That's because when you cut your carbs it takes a while for the hormones that regulate insulin secretion to catch on. Until they do, your pancreas pumps out the dose of insulin it has been using to cover the glucose your high carb diet was dumping into your bloodstream. When you cut off that supply of glucose, this excess insulin can push your blood sugar down to a very low level.

If you test your blood sugar with a meter while feeling shaky, you often will see a completely normal blood sugar. This is because when your blood sugar drops into the truly hypoglycemic range that poses a real threat to your brain's supply of glucose, your adrenals immediately release stress hormones that push your blood sugar back up again. They do this very quickly, so that by the time you start feeling shaky, the stress hormones have already pushed your blood sugar back up. But since these hormones *are* stress hormones, they will also get your pulse pounding and your heart thumping. Even after your blood sugar is back in the normal range, it can take an hour or more for these stress hormones to dissipate.

Another reason you might feel dizzy or shaky when you start a low carb diet is that the diet can lower your blood pressure. If you are taking blood pressure medications, you may need to adjust your dosage. If your blood pressure drops too low, that can also trigger the release of the same stress hormones that raise blood sugar out of the danger zone. Talk to your doctor or pharmacist about how to adjust the dose of your blood pressure medication safely. Some blood pressure medications can not be stopped suddenly without raising your risk of heart attack.

Though the low carb diet is very effective, long-term, at eliminating hunger, in the first few days of a low carb diet, you *will* feel surges of hunger if you experience low blood sugars caused by your body secreting more insulin than it needs. The hunger caused by true hypoglycemia can best be described as "the raving munchies." It's a gnawing, impossible to ignore kind of hunger that makes you want to drop everything and ransack the fridge.

Many people have heard that the best way to deal with hypogly-cemic attacks is to eat a piece of cheese or drink a glass of orange juice, but neither will correct the problem in a timely way. Cheese works too slowly. It can take up to 6 hours for the proteins in cheese to turn into carbohydrates and raise your blood sugar. If you eat cheese at meal time instead of high carb food, it will, of course, in long term lead to your having fewer attacks of low blood sugar, which is why doctors tell people to eat high protein snacks when they are hypoglycemic. But cheese won't calm the hunger arising from a hypoglycemic attack.

Orange juice is also a poor choice for countering hypoglycemia because it has too much sugar in it and will raise your blood sugar too much, which will stimulate a further insulin release and set off a rollercoaster of high and low blood sugars that will increase rather than decrease your hunger.

Most people will find that at the start of their diets, if they can just sit tight through a day or two of this kind of hypoglycemic response, it goes away. Usually our bodies reset how much insulin they secrete very quickly. However, people who are extremely insulin resistant and secrete huge amounts of insulin may need more time to adjust to a lower carb intake.

The Two Gram Cure

If after the first few days of your diet you still find yourself being overcome with a relentless attack of the munchies caused by plummeting blood sugars, one way to alleviate it is to eat a very small dose of pure glucose, one just big enough to raise your blood sugar 10 mg/dl.

The actual amount it will take to do this depends on your body weight. For a person who weighs around 150, two grams will do it. The table below shows the amount of glucose needed to eat to raise a person's blood sugar 10 mg/dl based on their weight

.

Weight	Glucose
140 lb	2 g
175 lb	2.5 g
210 lb	3 g
245 lb	3.5 g
280 lb	4 g
315 lb	4.5 g

You can get two grams of glucose from any candy whose primary sugar is dextrose, since dextrose is just another name for glucose. Five Smarties discs (the American kind, not the English ones) or one hard Sweetarts candy wafer of the kind that is sold in a roll at drugstore or quick stop checkout counters will do it. After you've taken the glucose, wait fifteen minutes. You should feel better and much less hungry. Do *not* repeat the two gram cure more than once a day. This is an emergency strategy, not an excuse to eat candy!

The two gram cure won't help with the ravenous hunger that can be caused by the fluctuating female hormones that cause PMS, which, as you may recall, may be related to the threefold rise in ghrelin many women experience a few weeks before menstruation. That kind of hunger doesn't respond to anything except the passage of time—though fortunately it usually only lasts a day or two. Knowing that nothing you can eat will make any difference in this particular kind of hunger may help you tough it out and not try to assuage it by eating.

Points to Remember from This Chapter:

1. Common side effects associated with low carb diets usually occur during the first weeks of the diet as the body adapts to lowered blood sugars.

2. Ketogenic diets have several additional side effects that occur as the brain switches to burning ketones or that result from the dehydration that occurs when glycogen is depleted.

3. A small sprinkle of potassium chloride can alleviate leg cramps, but it is only safe to use if you aren't taking potassium-sparing blood pressure medications

4. The ravenous hunger caused by low blood sugars early on in the diet can be limited by taking a few grams of pure glucose, once a day, when blood sugars are dropping too low.

Chapter 12
Supplements and Functional Foods

I receive a lot of emails from people who visit my Blood Sugar 101 web site asking which supplements they should take. This is no surprise. Drug stores, health food stores, and health-related web sites offer dozens of supplements that claim to lower blood sugar and speed weight loss. Diet books, too, promote supplements as if they had miraculous effects. The news media regularly publish studies funded by food manufacturers claiming common foods like chocolate or blueberries also have miraculous healing properties. Then companies market extremely expensive versions of these same foods at premium prices labeling them as "functional foods."

Why You Must Be Skeptical

Most of these claims are pure hype, and few supplements live up to them. The money to be made by selling supplements dwarfs the millions available to those, like Kimmer, who sell fraudulent diet plans. Supplements are completely unregulated in the United States. So anyone can sell you anything in a capsule, labeled any way they want, as long as they don't print a health claim on the label.

The only time a supplement maker will get investigated is if their supplement makes someone sick enough that their doctor reports it to the FDA. For this to happen, the doctor must link the use of the supplement to the subsequent illness. But this rarely happens. Few doctors would think that a Chinese herb might be the cause when a middle aged patient with high blood pressure develops kidney failure. And if you expensive supplement does *nothing*, you're out of luck. There's no legal requirement that the expensive supplements you buy must do anything. And most don't.

People embarking on low carb diets are flooded with ads for these miracle cures as soon as they visit any web site that discusses the diet. Because some objective-looking diet web sites are owned by companies that exist primarily to sell supplements and "health foods" dieters who visit discussion forums looking for information may be given "helpful" information by shills working for supplement sellers. These people pretend to be ordinary dieters who have experienced wonderful results taking this or that expensive supplement or miracle food.

People who post messages debunking the value of these supplements may abruptly vanish. That's because some of these web sites have a policy of blocking people's access if they don't support the web site owners agenda — which is to sell as many "low carb" products and supplements as possible.

The web is also full of web sites branded with the names of media-savvy physicians. These pop up at the top of the search page when you Google the supplements and appear to discuss their benefits in an objective manner. But their objectivity is suspect, because many of these sites also sell the doctor's own branded supplements, often with labels that make it impossible to know what exactly is in the pills they're pushing.

Web sites run by supplement manufacturers cite legitimate-looking research studies that turn out to have been paid for by the companies selling the products. Most of these studies have been published, if they were published at all, in "vanity journals" that will publish anything as long as the authors are willing to pay a hefty publication fee. Many of the vanity journals have titles that are similar to those of legitimate medical journals. So you have to stay alert.

The other problem with supplements is that even if they do work, because the U.S. supplement industry is completely unregulated, you have no way of knowing if the bottle you buy actually contains the supplement. When consumer groups occasionally take supplements to the lab for analysis, the reports can be eye-opening. For example, when taken to the lab, bottles supposedly containing the appetite suppressant hoodia were found to contain sawdust and the ground up root of the plant which is not chemically active. (Natural News: Hoodia) Several "natural" herbal mixtures sold for lowering blood sugar have been found, upon analysis, to contain doses of a very cheap generic sulfonylurea drug of the kind that is no longer prescribed in the U.S because it significantly raises the risk of heart attack.

And even if the supplement does contain what the label says it does, we know nothing about the long-term effects of most supplements, since studies of their efficacy rarely last more than a few weeks and rarely include control groups. We've learned from experience with prescription drugs, which are far more comprehensively tested before they enter the market, that it takes at least ten years for serious problems to emerge when people are taking a physiologically active substance every day. But only a tiny number of the hundreds of supplements you can buy have been studied for more than a few weeks. When long-term studies were performed for megavitamins, a generation after celebrity doctors had started promoting them, the results showed that these supplements appeared to raise, not lower, the risk of premature death.

Finally, though you may be told that herbal remedies are more "natural," strychnine is also natural, and herbs that have medical properties turn out to do so by affecting the same cellular pathways used by pharmaceutical drugs. For example, the traditional Chinese medicines bitter melon and ginseng both lower blood sugar, but they do so by affecting the same receptors as sulfonylurea drugs, which have been found to also raise the risk of heart attacks, because these same receptors are found in heart muscle. (Rotshteyn, 2004)

It is also possible to lower blood sugar by damaging the liver, which is why people nearing the end stage of alcoholism will often develop hypoglycemia. So it is quite possible that a supplement that lowers blood sugar or causes weight loss is doing it in a way that is harmful.

Given what you learned in the last chapter about what really causes insulin resistance, you should be particularly wary of herbs grown in countries where agricultural chemicals aren't regulated. A study published in 2011 titled, "Heavy metal and pesticide content in commonly prescribed individual raw Chinese Herbal Medicines" makes it clear what else you may be getting with your herbs. It explains, "... 231 samples (69%) with heavy metals and 81 samples (28%) with pesticides had contaminants that could contribute to elevated levels of exposure. Wild collected plants had higher contaminant levels than cultivated samples." (Harris, 2011)

With all this in mind, let's review what research has found to be true about the supplements that supposedly improve weight loss or blood sugar control, block carbs, or curb your cravings for sweets.

Vitamin D

Vitamin D is a hormone which has been embraced both by mainstream and alternative medicine as a panacea for everything that ails us. That's largely because Vitamin D levels have been found to be low in people who are seriously overweight and in those with a variety of diseases, including autoimmune conditions like Multiple Sclerosis and Type 1 diabetes.

Unfortunately, supplementing with Vitamin D does not appear to reverse any of these conditions, though there are hints that supplementing with Vitamin D *before* people experience an autoimmune attack may prevent them from developing an autoimmune disease. (Zipitis, 2008)

Because Vitamin D levels are also low in people who develop Type 2 diabetes, there has been speculation that Vitamin D might improve insulin sensitivity. But a study in which people who were insulin resistant and deficient in Vitamin D were given massive doses of Vitamin D that raised their blood levels of the hormone to well within the normal range found that it made no change in their blood sugars or insulin sensitivity when measured using a glucose tolerance test. (Kai, 2008) This finding was duplicated in a second placebo-controlled study of 61 participants given placebo, 100,000 IU or 200,000 IU of Vitamin D3. (Witham, 2010)

Though the Vitamin D made a very small difference in the research subjects' blood pressure—which was still too high after supplementation—the study found "Insulin resistance and glycosylated haemoglobin [A1C] did not improve with either dose of vitamin D3."

Furthermore, a study of 446 European subjects diagnosed with metabolic syndrome found no relationship between their blood concentrations of vitamin D and their insulin secretion or sensitivity. This suggests that the low vitamin D levels seen in people with diabetes are a result, not a cause of their blood sugar disorder. (Gulseth, 2010)

Supplementing with large doses of Vitamin D can be dangerous because too much Vitamin D can cause high blood calcium levels in people who take supplemental calcium or get a lot of calcium from eating dairy products. Though the books written by doctors who promote Vitamin D as a miracle cure assure you this isn't true, it is. Because my doctor recommended it, I took 2000 IU of Vitamin D3 every day for two years, only to see my blood pressure soar and my blood calcium levels rise to the very top of the normal range—a level that turns out to be associated with a higher risk of heart disease, probably because it makes it more likely that calcium will get deposited in your arteries.

Doctors are now reporting that rampant Vitamin D supplementation has caused a revival in what used to be a rare condition, Milk Alkali syndrome, which occurs when people develop extremely high blood calcium levels that can be fatal. (Patel, 2010) Megadoses of Vitamin D also have been found to be associated with the occurrence of 26% more fractures in a group of elderly women who were taking it to avoid osteoporosis. (Sanders, 2010)

If you supplement with Vitamin D, get your blood levels of this hormone checked periodically, and lay off the supplementation when your levels are solidly within the normal range. At the time when I began supplementing with Vitamin D my levels were already within the normal range. By the time my blood calcium had become dangerously high, my Vitamin D levels were 71% higher than what they'd been when I started supplementing, and the endocrinologist who had urged me to supplement with Vitamin D now tells me that doctors are starting to think that levels in the high 50 ng/ml range, where mine ended up, are *not* healthy.

Also be aware that Vitamin D levels are reported using two kinds of units. The ng/mL unit used in most U.S. labs gives a reading that must be multiplied by 2.6 to give the nmol/L value you see reported in many, but not all, research studies. Raising levels reported in mg/dl to the levels cited in research studies that use the nmol/L units will result in your having abnormally high, and possibly dangerous levels.

It is possible that Vitamin K2 can prevent the accumulation of calcium in the arteries caused by Vitamin D or reverse it. (Guyenet: K2) But why attempt to prevent the damage caused by one questionable, unregulated supplement by taking another? It makes more sense to monitor your Vitamin D levels and only supplement when they are low.

B Vitamins

People embarking on low carb diets are often advised to supplement with B vitamins because a grain-free diet can be low in these important vitamins. Low Thiamine (vitamin B1) has been found in people with diabetes, but it is not clear if the lack of the vitamin causes the condition or is *caused* by exposure to high blood sugars.

Some preliminary research suggested that supplementing with Vitamin B1 might be helpful in reversing diabetic kidney disease. Unfortunately, subsequent studies found that supplementing with a "Single tablet of B vitamins containing folic acid (2.5 mg/d), vitamin B6 (25 mg/d), and vitamin B12 (1 mg/d)" for 3 years was associated with a *faster* deterioration in kidney function and a doubling of stroke risk. (House, 2010)

This suggests very strongly that you'd do best to avoid megadoses of B-Vitamins and get your B vitamins from foods, rather than pills.

Some good sources of all the B vitamins that are compatible with low carb diets include spinach, sunflower seeds, ham, pork chops, broccoli, mushrooms, eggs, liver, oysters, clams, chicken breast, green beans, broccoli, spinach, and asparagus.

If you do supplement, keep the doses within the range of the recommended daily requirement and avoid vitamin supplements that provide two or three times that RDA.

Magnesium

An analysis of data from the Nurses' Health Study suggests that an increased intake of dietary magnesium corresponded with a reduced risk of diabetes. This result was echoed by a similar finding using data from The Women's Health Study. (Lopez-Ridaura, 2003 and Song, 2003) Adequate blood levels of magnesium have also been found to counter high blood pressure.

However, it is not clear whether the high blood magnesium levels found in healthy people are keeping their blood sugar control from deteriorating or are a marker showing that a person does not have the underlying conditions that cause diabetes. It's also possible that the reason some women have high magnesium levels is that they are eating a healthier diet rich in fresh vegetables, while those with low levels are eating diets heavy in chemical-laced fast foods and processed foods which promote insulin resistance.

Magnesium and calcium work together, and many magnesium supplements also contain calcium, as supplementing magnesium alone can lower calcium levels. However, if you are eating a lot of cheese on your low carb diet you will already be getting a lot of calcium, and there is accumulating evidence that over-supplementing calcium can result in excess calcium being deposited in your arteries. (Bolland, 2008)

The safest and healthiest way to get your magnesium is by eating the nuts and leafy green vegetables that you should already be eating as part of a healthy low carb diet. Plentiful amounts of magnesium also are found in premium chocolates with a high percentage of cocoa, which can be quite low in carbohydrate.

Before you supplement with pills containing high levels of magnesium, ask your doctor to run a test for magnesium the next time you have blood work done. If your blood magnesium level is in the normal range, don't supplement with high doses. Up to 350 mg a day in addition to the magnesium you get in food is considered safe.

Cinnamon

Cinnamon is often touted as lowering blood sugar and improving insulin resistance, based on research done in 1990 by a team led by Richard A Anderson at the Human Nutrition Research Center of the FDA. His team was testing foods for an insulin-enhancing effect as part of a series of studies and cinnamon was only one of several foods his team described as having an insulin-enhancing effect. Others included peanut butter and tuna fish. (Khan, 1990)

In 2006, when cinnamon was anointed "magical cure of the month," Dr. Anderson's research was heavily quoted. However, closer inspection of his team's very small studies revealed that cinnamon's supposedly favorable effect had been determined only by measuring fasting blood sugar, not insulin. Research using glucose tolerance tests that examined how cinnamon affected post-meal insulin levels was published with a title that says it all, "Cinnamon supplementation does not improve glycemic control in postmenopausal 2 diabetes patients." (Vanschoonbeek, 2006)

A further study didn't even confirm Dr. Anderson's claim that cinnamon improves fasting blood sugars. It randomly assigned people with Type 2 diabetes to take either capsules containing 500 mg of cinnamon or a placebo every day for three months. It found no differences in the groups' average levels of blood sugar, insulin, or cholesterol. (Blevins, 2007)

Contrary to the claims of companies selling very expensive versions of cinnamon, Dr. Anderson's research, which was the only research that suggested cinnamon had any impact, was performed using the cassia variety of cinnamon—the kind you can find at any grocery store. If you want to test it out, to see if it makes any difference for you, there's no harm in doing so.

Chromium

There was a flurry of excitement about chromium in the 1990s, after the same Dr. Anderson who got such impressive results with cinnamon reported that chromium supplementation could significantly improve glucose tolerance. (Anderson RA, 1998)

Studies conducted in India and China suggested that supplementing with chromium lowered blood sugar significantly. However, studies conducted with European and American populations did not show chromium having any such effect.

A subsequent review of chromium research by NIH statisticians concluded that chromium supplementation had no effect on glucose or insulin levels in non-diabetic people and that the evidence for an effect on people with diabetes was inconclusive. (Althuis, 2002)

Some researchers speculated that the results seen in the Chinese and Indian studies might have been due to these particular populations subsisting on mediocre diets that were deficient in chromium. The diets eaten by most people in the First World supplies more than enough chromium.

The safest approach to chromium supplementation—as is the case with most mineral supplementation—is to get chromium through the foods you eat. Foods rich in chromium that are compatible with a low carb diet are seafood, green beans, broccoli, nuts, and peanut butter, all of which also contain other helpful micronutrients. Eating foods that contain vitamin C, like berries or green pepper, may increase the absorption of dietary chromium.

L-Carnitine

L-Carnitine is another supplement highly touted for weight loss, based, apparently, on the results of a veterinary study conducted on obese cats. (Center, 2000) There is no credible research suggesting it has the same effect in humans.

One study compared a group of moderately obese post-menopausal women who took 2 grams of L-Carnitine for eight weeks while walking for 30 minutes, four times a week, with a control group who didn't take the supplement. The results for both groups were identical. Neither group lost weight. However five of the women taking the L-Carnitine had to discontinue it because it caused nausea or diarrhea. (Villani, 2000)

Conjugated Linoleic Acid

Conjugated linoleic acid (CLA) is a fat found in dairy products. In the late 1990s, rodent research suggested it might boost weight loss. The published studies looking at its effects on humans suggest that it makes almost no difference in their weight while worsening insulin resistance by boosting lipid oxidation and that it raises levels of markers of inflammation like CRP.

Only one study in humans found any hint of improved weight loss in those taking CLA compared to a placebo. In that study, a group of postmenopausal women lost, altogether, a puny 1.76 lbs over a period of 16 weeks, but they developed increased insulin resistance. (Raff, 2009)

In a group of obese men studied for four weeks, there was no difference in scale weight, though the group taking CLA lost 3 millimeters when an obscure measurement of the abdomen was used, the "sagittal abdominal diameter." (Risérus, 2001) Two other studies found that CLA had no impact on weight loss, one in a group of weight lifters and another in a group of obese men. (Kreider, 2002 and Risérus, 2002)

In return for this less than breathtaking weight loss, subjects in several of these studies experienced increased insulin resistance — measured by the highly reliable insulin clamp method — as well as a rise in markers of oxidative stress and inflammation.

It turns out that the CLA molecule occurs in three different isomers — isomers are versions of a molecule that share the same chemical formula but have a different structure. Because their structures are different, different isomers of the same chemical behave differently in our bodies.

Two of these studies investigated the effects of taking various CLA isomers. They compared what happened to dieters taking the mixture of CLA isomers that are found in commercially-sold supplements to the results in dieters taking only the isoform found in cow's milk.

Both studies found that the mix of isomers found in supplements caused unhealthy changes, including rises in CRP and Tumor Necrosis Factor, an indicator of inflammation. The isomers found in supplements also caused a rise in insulin resistance, which was elegantly measured by looking at the expression of the GLUT 4 gene. Insulin causes this gene to turn on in cells when it is working properly.

The form of CLA found in cow's milk did not produce these negative health effects, but it also didn't make any difference in the dieters' weight when compared to a placebo. (Raff, op cit and Risérus op cit.)

The reason the CLA you can buy as a supplement differs chemically from the kind you get in cow's milk is that it doesn't come from milk. It is synthesized in the lab by chemically processing safflower oil, which does not naturally contain CLA. Once the safflower oil has been turned into the supplement isomer of CLA it is very prone to oxidation. Oxidized fats are known to damage to our organs. (Lee, 2004)

If you are eating full fat yogurt or cheese, you will be getting a very small amount of the isomer of CLA that doesn't harm your body. There is slightly more CLA in milk from pasture-fed cattle collected in the spring than in milk collected at other times of year. However you would have to eat 42 ounces of cheese to get the same amount of CLA that was used in these studies. (Kim, 2009)

CLA isn't the only supplement where a cheaply manufactured isomer may have a very different effect on your body from that of the isomer found in expensive foods. And because supplement manufacturers aren't regulated, their claims about the purity or the origins of their supplements have to be taken with a grain of salt.

Coenzyme Q10

Coenzyme Q10 (CoQ10) is often prescribed for people who have been taking statins because statins deplete the level of CoQ10 found in the cell. CoQ10 also appears to play an important role in the processes within the mitochondria that lead to the burning of glucose. As you'll recall, people become insulin resistant when their mitochondria don't burn glucose properly. It's possible that the way statins lower CoQ10 has something to do with why they cause insulin resistance.

It's also possible that CoQ10 may be helpful to the subset of overweight people who are overweight because their mitochondria don't burn glucose properly. People who are born with a damaged mitochondrial gene that causes a form of diabetes do experience better outcomes with long-term CoQ10 supplementation. (Suzuki, 1998) However, research on the impact of CoQ10 on people with other forms of diabetes comes up with mixed findings.

A study conducted in 1999 gave 30 men with hypertension and insulin resistance a daily dose of 120 grams of CoQ10 in hydrosoluble gel form for 8 weeks. It lowered their blood pressure and dramatically dropped their fasting blood sugars—which would have actually been considered diabetic had the researchers been using the criteria now used to diagnose diabetes. After supplementation, their average insulin secretion during a glucose tolerance test was cut in half, while their average blood sugar dropped from almost-diabetic to almost completely normal. This would strongly suggest that CoQ10 had dramatically reduced their insulin resistance. (Singh, 1999)

However, another study, conducted with people diagnosed with Type 2 diabetes did not duplicate these results. After treatment with CoQ10, their average fasting blood sugar dropped only slightly and remained well within the range that causes complications. Their average A1C actually deteriorated slightly. This study used a higher dose, 200 mg a day. (Hodgson, 2002)

It is possible that differences in the form of CoQ10 used for supplementation explain these contradictory results, as some forms may be more bioavailable than others. Or perhaps lower doses are more effective than larger ones. CoQ10 also acts as an antioxidant and higher doses of other antioxidants have been found to be damaging, even when low doses are helpful. If you have higher than normal blood sugars, you can test for yourself whether this supplement does anything for you by testing your blood sugar with a blood sugar meter one hour after eating a food that usually raises your blood sugar. Test before you start the supplement. Then a week or two after starting it test your blood sugar again after eating the same food.

Antioxidant Vitamins

Years ago, some small scale studies suggested that the antioxidant vitamins C and E might help prevent heart disease, and some people still believe these vitamins help control insulin resistance. However, numerous studies have concluded that not only do these vitamins not prevent heart disease, but they appear to be harmful.

A February 2007 study found that antioxidant supplements seemed to *raise* the risk of death in those who took them. (Bjelakovic, 2007) Vitamin E was found in the Physicians Health Study to increase the risk of hemorrhagic stroke. (Sesso, 2008)

A rodent study gives insight into why this might be. It found that high doses of antioxidants may interfere with cellular processes in a way that *increases* insulin resistance and raises the risk of diabetes. It turns out that the presence of some by-products of oxidation, which antioxidants remove, are necessary for proper signaling within the mitochondria. (Loh, 2009)

Selenium

Selenium is a mineral which some small, mostly animal-based experiments suggested might lower blood sugar. However, a study published in July of 2007, which attempted to see whether long-term supplementation with selenium would prevent Type 2 diabetes discovered that it appeared to do just the opposite.

The study was conducted in people living in parts of the U.S. where selenium intake is low. None of the study subjects had diabetes at the outset of the study. After more than 7 years, those who took the selenium supplements developed *more* diabetes than those who did not. Not only that, but the more selenium a person had in their blood plasma, the more likely they were to develop diabetes. Strike selenium off your list of supplements unless you want to get diabetes. (Stranges, 2007)

Red Yeast Extract

Many people, rightfully concerned about the dangers of taking statin drugs, believe it is safer to take a supposedly "natural" supplement, red yeast extract.

Unfortunately, this extract, when it really contains red yeast extract—and not all pills sold as red yeast extract do—contains a molecule that, chemically, *is* a statin. If you take your statin in the unregulated supplement form you get to play "guess the dosage," since there is no guarantee that the dose of the statin contained in red yeast extract is the same from pill to pill.

Even worse, The FDA warned on Aug 10, 2007 that several brands of red yeast extract illegally contain the prescription statin, lovastatin, though, not surprisingly, they did not list lovastatin in their ingredient list. (Medscape: FDA)

Given that we've just learned that statins increase insulin resistance and dramatically raise the risk of developing diabetes, this is another supplement you'd do well to avoid.

Coconut Oil

Coconut oil is a Medium Chain Triglyceride (MCT). Animal research suggests MCTs might ramp up the rate at which our bodies burn fat, and web bulletin boards are full of people posting exaggerated claims that coconut oil ramps up their ability to lose weight. But there is very little human research on this topic, and what little there is was all conducted by teams led by one person, Marie-Pierre St-Onge. Nevertheless you will often see coconut oil promoted as a fat burning miracle in books, alternative health web sites, and online diet discussion boards.

A review of Ms. St-Onge's studies shows that they are fairly small and short in duration. Despite titles like "Medium-Chain Triglycerides Increase Energy Expenditure and Decrease Adiposity in Overweight Men" the actual weight loss study subjects experienced that can be attributed to eating MCTs is very small. In one of her studies, a group of men whose average weight was 192 lbs at the start of the month-long study lost .9 lbs more than a group eating olive oil. When subjects in these studies lost fat on diets with MCT, the fat lost tended to be subcutaneous fat.

However, it is important to consider the methodology used in these studies. The oil the participants ate was not coconut oil, but a special "functional oil" which contained a customized mixture of MCTs that contained very little pure coconut oil.

More importantly, this MCT oil was not *added* to these men's diet, it *replaced* olive oil or other fats, since the methodology used ensured that both groups studied were eating essentially the same caloric intake. This is an important point. (St-Onge, March 2003 and St-Onge, Sept. 2003)

In another St-Onge study, the subjects in one diet group ate a calorie restricted weight loss diet which included 10 grams a day of MCT in the form of the functional oil. The study confirmed that replacing other oils with the functional oil didn't worsen metabolic parameters, but it also showed that consuming the functional oil didn't make any significant improvements to the subjects' fasting blood sugar or their abnormally high fasting insulin. (St-Onge, 2008)

The participants in all these studies were eating diets that were high in carbohydrate, for example, in one the diet composition was reported as being 40% fat, 15% protein, and 45% carbohydrates. In fact, in one of St-Onge's studies, published in a high impact journal, it's reported that the subjects ate diets where, "Both diets contained 40% of energy as fat, 55% as carbohydrates, and 15% as protein. Since this adds up to 110%, it makes you wonder how carefully these peer-reviewed studies are reviewed. (St-Onge, Sept 2003)

If you decide to use coconut oil in your diet, be sure you use it to replace other fats not in addition to them. When people in the online low carb diet community have experimented with coconut oil, they have often reported that it stalled their weight loss or even caused weight gain. That may be because they have added it to their diets without eliminating an identical amount of other fats.

Vinegar

You'll also hear a lot of hype claiming that vinegar, particularly apple cider vinegar, can cure all human ills. It's routinely touted as a treatment for insulin resistance and high blood sugars.

One published study claims that ingesting 2 tablespoons of vinegar lowers fasting blood sugar. Unfortunately, when you look at the actual study you find that it lowered it by such a tiny amount as to be meaningless. A small group of people whose fasting blood sugars were above 137 mg/dl—a level well into the diabetic range—took two tablespoons of vinegar before bed each night and lowered their fasting blood sugars by a whopping 5 to 8 mg/dl. This left them with dangerously high fasting blood sugars still well over the level used to diagnose diabetes. The study only lasted 3 days, so we don't know whether this effect faded out when the regimen was continued, as is often the case with any treatment that makes minor changes in blood sugar. (White, 2007)

Another study by this same group of researchers took 8 normal people, 11 people diagnosed with insulin resistance, and 10 people with diabetes and fed them a meal containing 84 grams of carbohydrate, with and without 20 grams of apple cider vinegar. The vinegar made a very small difference in the very large rise in blood sugar experienced by the people with diabetes, dropping the average blood sugar peak about 18 mg/dl, though it was still almost twice as high as that of the normal people fed the same meal.

The problem with this study is that the blood sugar rise in the study subjects was only measured for one hour after eating. Since it's likely that the reason vinegar has an effect on blood sugar is because it slows the digestion of starches, it's very possible that the glucose that didn't show up in people's bloodstreams an hour after eating would have shown up later.[19]

This study has a bit more credibility in that it did test vinegar against a placebo and used a glucose tolerance test that also measured insulin levels. So it suggests that vinegar may delay the digestion of starch for a short while, but it is very unlikely that it is actually improving insulin sensitivity as the authors claim. (Johnston, 2004)

You can test vinegar safely on your own. Don't use more than two tablespoons of vinegar with a single meal and if you develop stomach pain, stop.

Starch Blockers

Over-the-counter products made out of an extract of white kidney beans claim to be able to block the digestion of starch and allow you to consume carbohydrates without having them affect your blood sugar. They do this, they claim, by inhibiting the action of an enzyme called alpha amylase.

The company that makes these products lists a number of clinical studies on their web site that supposedly prove their products' effectiveness. These studies are all funded by the company selling the starch blockers. One, published in *The Open Neutraceuticals Journal*, displays charts that suggest that the starch blocker might decrease the amount of a white bread similar to Wonder Bread that got digested, but it also shows that it made a very small difference in how high blood sugar spiked after eating a mixed meal. (Vinson, 2009)

Though there isn't any independent research published about this product, there are prescription drugs that block the digestion of starch, and we know a bit more about them. One is acarbose, which is sold under the brand name Precose. According to the FDA-approved prescribing information for Precose, it is "... designed to slow down the actions of alpha-amylase and alpha-glucosidase enzymes thereby slowing the appearance of sugar in the blood after a meal."

Peer-reviewed studies have shown that people with diabetes who take acarbose lower their blood sugars very slightly. No study showed that taking acarbose caused any increase in weight loss. When I took Precose for several months I found it allowed me to add an additional 10 to 15 grams of carbohydrate to an otherwise very low carb meal without experiencing a blood sugar spike.

---

[19] Acids, wine, fatty acids, and fiber all slow digestion, but the slowed carbohydrates do eventually digest and when they do, they will raise blood sugar. (Dubois, 1985)

However, this kind of starch blocking is not a good solution for someone wanting to boost their carbs so they can eat normal food in social situations, because the most common side effects of *any* drug that slows or blocks starch digestion is intense, and, at times, intolerable, gas and diarrhea. That's because when starches and sugars pass into the intestine undigested they encounter a whole ecosystem of bacteria and yeast that *can* digest them.

They do this via fermentation and one of the end products of fermentation is carbon dioxide—the gas that makes your beer fizzy. Unfortunately, when it is produced by the microorganisms that ferment starches in your gut, the result is not fizziness but something far more explosive. Flatulence is listed in the official Precose prescribing information as occurring in 74% of those who took the drug.

Rumor has it that so many people had severe gastrointestinal reactions to Precose when it was first introduced that the company that makes it stopped its ad campaign and abandoned marketing it. Though it is still on the market, very few doctors prescribe it. Some people who have experimented with it have found that taking Beano, an over-the-counter supplement that helps people eat beans without producing gas, eliminates this side effect. Unfortunately, it does so by providing *other* enzymes that digest starch, which defeats the purpose of a starch blocker.

It isn't likely that the over-the-counter starch blocker is any more effective than Precose since it only inactivates one of the two enzymes Precose blocks. If it does lead to increased weight loss, as the manufacturer-paid research claims it does, it probably does so because those who take it quickly learn that the only way to avoid becoming a walking sewer-gas factory is to cut down dramatically on their starch intake. It is also possible that the digestive discomfort it causes decreases appetite.

If you take any of these starch blockers you need to be aware than none of them block the digestion of simple sugars.

Gymnema Sylvestre

Gymnema Sylvestre is an herb used in Aryuvedic and Chinese medicine. It appears to lower blood sugar, and claims are made that it lowers sugar cravings.

Unfortunately, most of the research investigating this herb is rodent research, which is often misleading because rodent blood sugar control works very differently from that of humans. That's why the press has reported hundreds of times that diabetes has been "cured" in mice though there's never been a hint of a cure that works in humans.

As is the case with so much research on supplements, most of the studies on this supplement were conducted in the Third World and published in obscure journals. This suggests it is vanity research commissioned by companies that sell the supplement. The most enthusiastic report touting the effects of Gymnema Sylvestre was published only in a newsletter run by the authors of the study, though it must be said that their newsletter is considered a reputable source for information about diabetes.

What peer-reviewed research I can find that explores the mechanisms by which this herb might work suggests that it increases insulin secretion and blocks the action of the same starch-digesting enzymes that Precose and the over-the-counter starch blockers block. (Persaud, 1999 and Ramkumar, 2010) Because this herb increases insulin secretion, it may be a poor choice for people who are insulin resistant who are already secreting higher than normal amounts of insulin.

Points to Remember from This Chapter:

1. Be suspicious of all claims made about supplements and functional foods as the research they are based on is often of poor quality or tainted by having been commissioned by companies selling the product.

2. Many supplements promoted as increasing weight loss, if they work at all, make only a tiny difference in the amount of weight lost, which doesn't justify their price.

3. Vitamins, minerals and trace substances can be dangerous when dosed in higher quantities than are found in food. Getting these nutrients from real food is the safest approach.

4. Supplements may be chemically the same as something that occurs in nature but when synthesized cheaply in the lab they may occur in the form of an unnatural isomer which has harmful effects on the body.

5. No supplement currently touted as lowering blood sugar does so in a way that makes any significant difference in health.

6. Starch blockers may limit the digestion of some starches, but these starches will still be fermented in the gut, which causes gas.

Chapter 13
Stalls

The data provided by lab researchers hints that something changes two months into most low carb diets, since that is when the average weight loss of the group slows down after a dramatic start. Six months in, the research shows that weight loss slows again. Messages posted on online support groups over the years give us additional insight into what is actually happening at these times when weight loss slows.

One of the most common kinds of posting you will see on any diet support group is one headed, "Help! I'm not losing." When the dieter has been on the diet for only a few weeks, the reason they think they've stalled is often because they have become so used to stepping on the scale each morning and seeing another pound gone that when a few days go by and the scale doesn't move they assume something is wrong.

You now know that this swift initial weight loss is caused primarily by the loss of glycogen and its associated water and that once glycogen is fully depleted all subsequent weight loss must come from burning off the body's fat stores, which will occur at a much slower rate. But after days or as weeks of losing discernable amounts each day, the slow rate at which fat burns off may make it feel like weight loss has completely stopped.

So many dieters, who think they have stalled, haven't. They are losing between .14 and .28 pounds of fat a day, which adds up to a pound or two a week. But these amounts are so small, they are impossible to detect amid the normal weight fluctuations that occur from day to day for other reasons.

Factors That Cause Weight Fluctuations

Here is a brief list of the factors that cause everyone's weight to vary from day to day by anywhere from one to five pounds:

1. The weight of the undigested food you ate during the day, which remains in your gut for 24 hours.

2. Water lost in breathing while you sleep. This water we give off in our breath is a product of respiration—a word that means breathing but also refers to the chemical reactions that occur in

our mitochondria which turn glucose and fat into carbon dioxide and water. We get rid of both each time we exhale. This may explain why most of us weigh less when we wake up than at any other time in the day.

3. How much sodium you ate the previous day. Most of the sodium we eat comes not from the salt shaker, but is hidden in processed foods and restaurant meals. A bigger than usual dose of sodium can make your scale weight soar the day after you've eaten it, adding anywhere from 2 to 4 pounds at once.

    It may take two more days for that sodium-related weight to disappear as your body rids itself of the sodium. Remember that many foods that are very high in sodium do not taste salty, including those full of MSG.

4. Stress hormones. The kind of stress we are taking here is not the kind that comes from the slow grinding misery of daily life but the kind that gets your heart pounding. These hormones increase your blood pressure by making your body hold onto sodium which can push up your weight, too.

    Going to the gym and doing a hard workout can cause you to secrete bursts of stress hormones, which can also slightly raise your blood sugar no matter what you ate. This is particularly true if you aren't eating a ketogenic diet and still have glycogen stored in your liver.

How to Detect Real Weight Loss

With so many factors contributing to daily weight fluctuations, the best way to determine if you are really stalled is to note your weight each day, ideally at the same time of day, since our weight rises over the course of the day. Average your daily weigh-ins once a week by adding up all 7 daily weights and dividing the total by 7. That's your weekly average weight.

If your average weekly weight this week is less than your average weekly weight from the previous week, you're losing weight. Average four weekly weights at the end of the month to get an average monthly rate. If this month's average weight is less than last month's, you aren't stalled.

How to Break a Stall

If your weight loss really has come to a screeching halt, especially early on in your low carb diet, there are several strategies that can help get it going again.

Weigh and Measure

The number one reason that people stop losing weight on their low carb diets is that they aren't actually eating a low carb diet.

If you've been cutting down on carbs by cutting out foods you know contain starches and sugars, like bread, cookies, and cake, you may still be getting a lot of carbohydrate from foods you thought were safe like salad dressing. For example, a single serving of Arby's "Fresh Market" Raspberry vinaigrette salad dressing contains 18 grams of carbohydrate, 16 grams of it in the form of sugar. This is almost as much as you'd get in a slice of bread.

There are carbs in quite a few restaurant foods you wouldn't expect to contain carbohydrate, too. For example, the "meat" in Taco Bell's tacos contains flour. And nacho cheese sauce may have a lot of starch filler.

Even if you've been checking what's in your food by diligently reading the labels, the portion size given for most foods on labels and in nutritional databases is often much smaller than what a reasonable person would consider an actual portion.

For example, the nutritional information on most cans of Campbell's soup give nutritional information based on a portion size that assumes you get 2.5 servings from the can. But most people get 2 servings out of that same can. So the nutritional information has underestimated the content of your real world portion by 20%. And though 6 is the usual number of portions listed on the label for standard sized jars of spaghetti sauce, when did you ever get six servings from a single bottle?

This portion size problem affects almost everything listed in nutritional databases. The sugar-free muffins sold at my supermarket, for example, list their nutritional information based on a portion size of 2 ounces. Since the carb count given on the muffin label for a single serving is 21 grams, it would be easy to think that half a muffin would fit well into even a very low carb diet plan. But it turns out the whole muffin weights not 2 oz but *5 oz*, so if you ate half of that muffin you'd have packed away 26 grams of carb, not 10, a significant difference. Make that kind of mistake a few times a day and your low carb diet is no longer low in carbs.

That's why the food scale is the most powerful tool you have for combating stalls. Use it along with a software tool that logs your exact food intake throughout the day and you are likely to discover why you've stalled.

You can buy a very good food scale for around $25. Food logging software can be found free on `http://fitday.com`.

You can also download "try before you buy" nutritional software from:

`http://www.calorieking.com`

or

`http://LifeForm.com`

There are also an ever increasing number of smartphone apps like Calorie Counter, Myfitnesspal, Low Carb Diet Assistant, and CarbsControl, which you can download. These can give you nutritional counts for the food you are eating and will track your daily intake. Some even scan your plate and estimate portion size, though you should test these estimates at home using your food scale before you rely on them.

Once you have bought a scale, dedicate a day when you are home all day to learning about the portion sizes of the foods you usually consume. Weigh everything you eat that day on your food scale and put the results into your food logging software. Track every mouthful all day long. You may be astonished to learn how different what you are actually eating is from what you thought you were eating.

If you have to eat out a lot, bring portions home and weigh them. Most fast foods and restaurant foods are served in portions that can be significantly larger than the sizes listed on the restaurants' web site.

In general, it's a good idea to avoid restaurants entirely when your weight loss has stalled because when you eat out it is so difficult to estimate what you are really eating. The immense portions many restaurants serve also make it easy to overeat. And that doesn't even get into the issue of how likely you are to find tempting high carb accompaniments served with whatever you order.

One handy tip: if you *do* get served more food than you should eat or if your restaurant plate shows up with an unexpected and tempting high carb side dish, sprinkle the food you don't want to eat with salt and pepper. This is a lot more effective than willpower. Though many of us have been conditioned not to waste food, it's better to waste food that will make you fat and unhealthy than to eat it.

Eliminate "Low Carb" Foods that Aren't Low in Carbs

If you've been eating foods labeled as being "low carb," especially those that use the phrase "Net carbs" somewhere on the label, you may be consuming far more carbohydrate than you realize.

Food manufacturers sell many foods that claim to be perfect for low carb diets. Many list appealingly low carb counts on the front of the package along with the phrase, "Net carb," making it sound like the product only contains 2 or 3 grams of carbohydrate. Often their ingredient lists contain mysterious substances like maltitol, glycerine, polydextrose, and resistant starch. But the actual carb count on the back of the package, where the FDA-mandated nutrition panel appears, lists far more grams of carbohydrates than the "net carbs" you see on the front.

Food companies claim these substances have a "negligible effect on blood sugar" but on September 26, 2002, Atkins Nutritionals, Inc. settled a class action suit and was assessed a fine because the labels of its Advantage Bars had mislead buyers by not including the 20+ grams of glycerine in the bars in the carbohydrate section of the bars' nutritional panel. (LCF: Settlement)[20]. Glycerine is metabolized as a carbohydrate when people are eating ketogenic diets and many people with diabetes, myself included, who tested their blood sugar with meters had found that these supposedly low carb bars sent their blood sugar skyrocketing.

After that, Atkins Nutritionals came up with the "Net Carbs" designation it now places on the front of wrappers along with the statement that the other carbs the nutritional label lists can be ignored. This ruse was so successful, other companies have adopted it. This is why so many foods marketed today as "low carb" aren't.

Sugar Alcohols

Sugar alcohols are the substances whose carbohydrate content is most frequently ignored when companies come up with deceptive "net carb" counts. Despite wrapper claims to the contrary, sugar alcohols *are* metabolized. That's why US law requires that they be reported as carbohydrates on nutritional labels and why their calories are included in calorie counts.

---

[20] The actual text of this settlement was posted on the Atkins Nutritionals, Inc. web site for several years. The fine was merely a slap on the wrist. In order for people who had been deceived by the packaging to share in the cash settlement, they had to have proof they had bought the bars several years before. Understandably, very few people had retained the receipts or used wrappers that would have made them eligible.

Despite their name, these substances aren't sugars or alcohols. They are hydrogenated starch molecules, which are a byproduct of corn processing. These sugar alcohols are manufactured by the three large agribusiness companies: SPI Polyols, Roquette America, Inc. and Archer Daniels Midland—the same companies that saturated the world with high fructose corn syrup. Hydrogenating corn starch molecules is yet another way to wring profits out of surplus corn.

Different sugar alcohols digest into 1 to 3 calories worth of glucose depending on which one you choose. Erythritol contains the fewest calories, delivering less than one calorie per gram. Maltitol—the most common sugar alcohol found in "low carb" and "sugar free" foods—contains the most, delivering 3 calories per gram. That is only one calorie less than 4 calories you find in table sugar and regular starch. What this means is that each gram of Maltitol contains .75 grams of carbohydrate.

People with diabetes who use blood sugar meters find that Maltitol can have a very significant impact on blood sugar. My blood sugar rose almost as high when I tested a serving of maltitol-sweetened Russell Stover "No Sugar" candy as it did when I ate a serving of the same size of regular Russell Stover candy. The only difference was that the "no sugar" candy took two hours to raise my blood sugar, not one—and tasted nasty.

But it isn't just people with diabetes who will experience this effect. A comprehensive review published by the Canadian *Journal of Diabetes* cites research that shows that chocolate bars sweetened with maltitol raised the blood sugar of *normal* people as high as did chocolate bars sweetened with table sugar. (Wolever, 2002)

There *are* successful low carb dieters who report that they have been able to lose significant amounts of weight while eating low carb treats filled with sugar alcohols every day. This may be due to one of two possible explanations. One is that they can lose weight eating more carbohydrate than they think they can. The other is that some people may lack an enzyme needed to digest sugar alcohols, which would let them pass through their guts largely undigested.

Lending some support to this idea is the fact that some of the people who report that they don't experience a blood sugar rise when they eat sugar alcohols experience intense diarrhea or gas later on. These are classic symptoms of what happens when starches pass undigested into lower gut where they may be fermented by bacteria (causing gas) or suck water out of cells lining the colon (causing diarrhea).

Resistant Starch

Resistant starches are another questionable ingredient found in foods marketed to low carb dieters. One brand of pasta lists 41 grams of carbohydrate on the official nutritional label, but elsewhere on the package claims it only delivers 5 grams of "digestible carbs" per serving.

In January of 2011 someone took this pasta to the lab and came up with definitive proof of what many of us with diabetes had found to be true, anecdotally. They published a research paper in a high impact diabetes journal that showed that this supposedly "low carb" pasta produced a glucose curve identical to that of regular pasta.

I blogged about this study when it was published. However, you can't read that study because the authors were forced to retract it—not because the data were flawed—but "because some of the data were obtained prior to receiving IRB [Institutional Review Board] approval." (Nuttall, 2011)

IRBs are set up to protect the public from unethical research. It's possible that the institution the authors of this study work retracted their study because they had committed a horrifying ethical violation by forcing innocent volunteers to eat pasta, but it is just as likely that the institution came up with this excuse to force the authors to retract an otherwise accurate study because they didn't have the deep pockets needed to withstand a lawsuit launched by the manufacturer of a highly profitable product that costs more than twice as much as regular pasta though it is, in fact, regular pasta.

Cheap regular pasta releases its carbohydrates very slowly over 4 or 5 hours, which is why nutritionists often suggest people with diabetes eat it. However, all those grams of carbohydrate do digest into glucose over time and when they do they will raise the blood sugar of people whose insulin isn't working properly.[21]

Misleading Fiber Counts

Most fiber, unlike sugar alcohols, is not metabolized and does not turn into blood sugar. Therefore some low carb authors tell you that fiber can be safely deducted from the total carb count given on a food's official nutritional label.

Unfortunately, this is no longer always true. Labeling laws outside United States treat fiber differently than do U.S. laws, and in many European countries. Fiber, though listed as a separate line item under "total carbohydrate," is *already* deducted from the official nutritional

---

[21] Fresh pasta, the kind that is not sold in dried form, can digest very quickly as it isn't made out of durum wheat. In that case, it raises blood sugar quite high very fast.

label's total carb count. This means that you can't deduct the 3 grams of fiber found on the nutritional label of imported Scandinavian bran crackers from the 3 grams of total carbohydrate listed on the same label. These crackers do *not* contain zero grams of carbohydrate. If they followed U.S. labeling conventions, their labels would show 6 grams of carbohydrate and 3 grams of fiber. But the European labels have already deducted the fiber from the total carb count. This is also true of many imported chocolates.

Over the past decade, many products that are made by U.S. companies have taken to deducting fiber from their total carb counts, too. For example, despite the fact that most labels for walnuts usually list 3 grams total carbohydrate and 3 grams fiber, walnuts are not a zero carb treat. This habit of listing total carbohydrates with the fiber already deducted has spread to many common foods like squash and beans that are hardly premium European imports

If you have any doubt about whether to deduct fiber, a simple solution is this. Use a hidden carb calculator. There are many on the web including some freeware ones you can download to your computer. The Low Carb Diet Tools - Hidden Carbs Calculator can be found at:

http://www.lowcarb.ca/low-carb-tools/hidden_carbs.html

Plug in the data from your label, and if the actual carb count is higher than the stated count, assume the label has already deducted the fiber carbs.

Don't Overdo Proteins

Another common reason people stall on ketogenic low carb diets is because they are eating too much protein. Excess protein not only raises your insulin levels but it can turn into glucose and raise your blood sugar. So just remember that by the time your daily carbohydrate intake has risen to 60 grams a day, unless you're playing football or doing a very intense body building regimen you probably don't need to eat any more protein than the usual amount it takes to repair and maintain your body tissues. For many of us this will work out to barely half a gram per pound of our body weight. You already learned how to calculate your protein in Chapter 11. If you are eating more than the protein calculator suggests, cut back.

Calories count

Some people are stalled because, though they are eating low carb, they aren't eating a diet. If you are eating more calories than you burn, you aren't going to lose weight, no matter what the composition of your diet.

It's possible to be in a highly ketogenic state for weeks, spilling enough ketones in your urine to turn ketone-detecting strips deep purple each morning, and still not lose a pound. This is a common experience among dieters who have been on a ketogenic diet for more than a few weeks, and one that has even been documented in a study titled, "Urinary ketones reflect serum ketone concentration but do not relate to weight loss in overweight premenopausal women following a low-carbohydrate/high-protein diet." (Coleman, 2005)

All ketones in your urine prove is that you are burning fat. It doesn't tell you where that fat comes from. So if you are eating enough fat to provide all the energy your body needs, your cells will burn that dietary fat and leave your body fat stores unchanged.

So once you've made sure you are eating only as much carbohydrate as you thought you were, and after you've cut back on excess protein, if you're still stalled, it's time to cut down on your calories. There are some fortunate people who are able to lose a lot of weight on a low carb diet without ever thinking about calories. But if you are stalled after following the steps we've just outlined, you have just learned you are not one of them.

Even people who start out their diet able to eat whatever they please without considering calories often find that, as they get closer to a normal weight, calories start to play a role. That's because the number of calories it takes to maintain your weight decreases as that weight drops. A 300 lb woman can lose weight eating 600 more calories a day than a woman can eat who weighs 200 lbs. But with each 25 pounds she loses, the number of calories that once-300 lb woman dieter must eat each day to keep on losing drops by about 150.

Age matters too, because our metabolisms slow with each passing year. Most women find that it's very tough to lose weight after menopause unless they carefully watch their calories.

Because bestselling diet books have sold the low carb diet to the public with the promise that it frees them from the tyranny of having to count calories, many low carb dieters who stall blame their stalls on excess carbs and attempt to break these stalls by cutting out the 10 or 15 grams a day of carbohydrates they were getting from green vegetables.

This is foolish. Cutting the 6 grams of carb you'll find in seven ounces of green beans with its 36 calories is not going to make the difference in your weight that you can make by cutting the 6 grams of carbs you get from eating 6 ounces of cheddar cheese—because those carbs are accompanied by an additional *720 calories*. I've even seen people suggesting that it was the 7 grams of "hidden carbs" in a cup of cream that stalled their diet, rather than the 820 calories that crea contributed.

Overly carb-centric thinking leads low carb dieters to come up with some very questionable explanations as to why high calorie foods stall them. Some decide they are "sensitive" to dairy, because when they eliminate the cups of cream and blocks of cheese that have been the mainstay of their diet their weight starts to drop, as it will when you remove all those hundreds of calories from your daily diet.

Others blame a "sensitivity" to pork, because they start losing when they stop snacking on pork rinds that contain 160 calories per ounce or stop eating half a pound of bacon every day which eliminates 1,200 calories.

While some low carb dieters may find that they can maintain their weight on a ketogenic low carb diet while eating more calories than they can eat on other diets without gaining, most of us will have to eat less fat than our bodies burn each day to burn off the excess poundage stored in our body's fat deposits.

Eliminate Artificial Sweeteners

One of the most interesting scientific discoveries of the late 2000s was that we have taste receptors sensitive to sweet tastes in both our gut and in our brain. These receptors are similar, if not identical, to those found in the taste buds on our tongues. Unlike glucose receptors, which ignore artificial sweeteners, these taste receptors respond to *any* chemical that your taste buds would taste as sweet, so they respond to calorie-free artificial sweeteners including sucralose, aspartame, and stevia.

When these taste receptors in your gut and brain sense sweetness, your brain assumes that glucose is on its way and sends out signals that stimulate your pancreas to secrete insulin. Since no glucose is actually coming in, this insulin will push your blood sugar down below its baseline level, which stimulates hunger. (Ren, 2009 and Sclafani, 2007)

This finding gives credence to research and anecdotal reports that foods and sodas containing artificial sweeteners increase how much people eat. This finding also ends the endless discussions about which artificial sweetener is best. As far as these sweet-sensing taste buds in your brain and stomach are concerned, it won't matter if the nonnutritive sweetener you use is natural or lab-created—the fact that it tastes sweet will cause the small insulin release that may lower your blood sugar and make you hungrier.

If you have been consuming a lot of artificial sweetener, it might be helpful to cut out all artificial sweeteners for a few weeks. When you do, you'll upregulate your sweet receptors and find that many unprocessed foods that didn't used to taste sweet have developed a sweet taste, particularly vegetables. By the same token, commercially sweetened food will taste overwhelmingly sugary.

After you've reset the sensitivity levels of your sweet sensors, you may find that you can achieve just the right amount of sweetening for the occasional food that could use it, by adding only half a teaspoon of real sugar—2 grams' worth. The sweetness of small amount of real sugar will affect your gut and brain exactly the way that the brain expects it to and may be more satisfying than an artificial sweetener—besides tasting better.

Get your Iron Level Checked

Though we all know that too little iron causes anemia, which leaves us feeling exhausted, few people realize that having too *much* iron in our bodies is even more dangerous. That's because high levels of iron damage various organs, including the heart, brain, and the pancreas. When iron damages the pancreas it can result in elevated blood sugars, and there is some evidence that the higher the body's iron stores, the more insulin resistant a person becomes.

There's also some evidence that people with abnormally high blood iron levels are more apt to have heart attacks. (Fernández-Real, 2002) Ten to 15% of people of European ancestry carry one gene for hemochromatosis, a condition in which the body accumulates very high iron stores. People who have inherited two genes develop the full-fledged disease, where high levels of iron are deposited in their organs. This usually doesn't cause symptoms until middle age, when they are likely to develop diabetes, joint pain, and liver damage. However, people who carry only one gene may also have higher than normal iron stores, which contribute to insulin resistance. If you have one of these genes, a low carb diet that is very high in red meat may be making your blood sugars worse because it is raising your blood iron levels, and this may contribute to a stall.

The test doctors use to check for these higher than normal iron stores is the ferritin test. If it returns a higher than normal value, you should cut back on your intake of red meat, and avoid cooking in cast iron pans. It would also be a good idea to avoid all multivitamins that contain iron. Because vitamin C also increases iron storage, if your iron level is high, don't take supplemental Vitamin C. High iron is usually more of a problem for men than women until menopause. Giving blood can also lower your ferritin level temporarily. (Berkeley Wellness Letter, 2004)

When Nothing Works

If you are still stalled after trying all these suggestions, one of two things is true. Either you have an undiagnosed metabolic problem that requires the help of a skilled endocrinologist, or you have, without realizing it, reached goal.

Get Help with Undiagnosed Medical Conditions

Some of the endocrine problems that can cause weight gain are undiagnosed thyroid disease, including marginal thyroid disease that cannot be diagnosed accurately with the tests most family doctors run, severe insulin resistance, PCOS (polycystic ovary syndrome), Cushing's disease, and certain unusual brain conditions. The kinds of diabetes and prediabetes that are caused by having beta cells that don't produce normal amounts of insulin or that are dying from an autoimmune attack can also raise your blood sugars to levels that cause hunger, even when you are eating a very low carb diet.

There are medications that can help all of these conditions. The hard part is finding a good endocrinologist who is willing to give you the tests and treatment you need. You will do best seeing endocrinologists who practice out of high quality teaching hospitals. These are the big city hospitals that are associated with medical schools. If you can't find a good endocrinologist, research the conditions you might have online and visit support groups for these conditions to learn what tests will give you the information you need to get an accurate diagnosis. Then go to your family doctor and demand those tests.

If you need to consult a doctor to help you with a blood sugar problem, *eat a high carb diet for two weeks before you take any medical tests.* Strange though it seems, most doctors have no idea how dramatically a low carb diet lowers blood sugar levels. If you take the blood tests they order while you are eating a low carb diet, you will almost certainly get back test results that look so normal the doctor will refuse to treat you. This happens even to people who have previously been diagnosed with diabetes.

In the past it was possible to get numbers that would make a doctor take you seriously, just by carbing up for a few days. But with doctors now universally using the A1C test to screen for diabetes, you run the risk of getting normal numbers if you have only carbed up for a few days before your lab visit, even if you have full-fledged diabetes.

So to get an A1C value that will convince a doctor that you need help with your blood sugars, you will have to let your blood sugars rise to the unhealthy levels they reach when you aren't eating a low carb diet. Let them remain there for the two weeks it takes to produce a convincing A1C test result. Once you've been to the doctor, go back to cutting the carbs.

Treating thyroid disease, PCOS, insulin deficiency, or extreme insulin resistance with safe, appropriate medications often will get weight loss going again when diet alone has failed. If you turn out not to be making normal amounts of insulin, don't be afraid to inject it. Those of us who are insulin deficient may find it easier to lose weight once insulin injections flatten our blood sugars because that will keep us from being hungry all the time.

People with Type 2 diabetes who complain that they started to gain weight when they started injecting insulin are almost always the victims of doctors who prescribe one-size-fits-all insulin regimens that don't match insulin doses to their carbohydrate intake. Insulin prescribed correctly should flatten blood sugars and eliminate hunger. If you need to use insulin, research the proper way to dose it by reading up on the subject. The book, *Dr. Bernstein's Diabetes Solution*, is a very good place to start, even if you eat more carbohydrate than he prescribes.

You May Have Reached Your Weight Loss Goal

If you've been dieting for a year or more, carefully watching your intake to be sure you're eating what you want to be eating, and have already lost 20% or more of your starting weight, a prolonged stall may your body's way of telling you that you've reached the only weight loss goal that you will be able to successfully maintain. This is particularly true if you are already limiting your calories to the point where cutting them down any further would push you over the line that distinguishes "careful eating" from "starvation."

Most people who stick to a low carb diet find they are able to lose that first 20% without feeling deprived. But to break through the very common stall that kicks in past that point, you may have to cut back on calories so severely that your body will decide you are starving and safety systems that have evolved over millions of years of mammalian life will kick in to make sure that you don't.

If that happens, you may have to live for years, or even the rest of your life, with a metabolism that has only one major goal—to get back that big chunk of the weight you just took off. Some solid research done at clinics where people have worked with doctors to lose 100 lbs or more suggests that people who have achieved very large weight losses have slower metabolisms than others, though other research addressing this topic comes to conflicting conclusions.

Some studies have found that dieting doesn't slow people's metabolic rate. But other studies hint that people who become severely overweight may have been born with slower than normal metabolisms, so while their metabolisms may not slow down when they diet, even when they remain at the same rate as usual, that rate is still slower than normal.

Some very high quality research that addresses this question was conducted at Rockefeller University at a clinic run by one of the grand masters of metabolic research, Rudolf Liebel. His clinic has been treating extremely obese people for over twenty years in an in-patient, highly controlled environment where they use sophisticated tools to measure exactly how much energy their subjects burn. Researchers at his clinic careful measured the metabolic rates of pairs of people who weighed the same amount. In each pair, one person had dieted down to that weight from a much higher weight and the other had never weighed more than it.

His study found that the people who had dieted down to the weight burned significantly less energy than the people of the same weight who had never dieted. More importantly, it found that these changes persist "regardless of whether that reduced weight has been maintained for weeks or years." (Rosenbaum, 2008)

These studies underline the fact that the larger the weight loss you achieve, the less you will be able to eat when you are maintaining. More to the point, when you stall, you have just hit the point where *you are maintaining your current weight.*

Taking off more weight will not only require that you eat less now, it will require that you eat less forever after if you want to maintain any further gains. Though many dieters imagine that once they reach goal, they'll be able to stop dieting and eat a lot more food, this is almost never true. Many of us find that once we reach goal, even on a low carb diet we can only eat another 200 or 300 calories a day above what we were eating during the month before we lost our last pound.

With that in mind, when you experience a prolonged stall, no matter how much more you might want to lose, it might be a very good idea to stop dieting and see if you can maintain your *current weight* before you do anything to try to take off more.

The other benefit of going into maintenance mode for a few months, even when you have more weight left you'd like to lose, is that it will let you figure out exactly how much more food you can eat when you *aren't* dieting for weight loss.

From a health standpoint, there is no reason not to pause once you've achieved a loss of more than 10% of your starting weight, since most research suggests that losing only that much is enough to give us the health benefits of weight loss. But as we've seen, those health benefits evaporate if we mismanage maintenance.

So stopping to ensure that you can maintain is a very healthy thing to do, especially if you plan to raise your carbs. If you practice raising your carbs and cutting back on your fat intake for a few months now and then *before* you reach goal, you might make it possible to avoid the dangerous mistakes that make some low carb diets very unhealthy over long term, no matter how much weight dieters lost.

Even if you end up heavier than you might wish, if you can maintain the weight loss you've already achieved for 5 years, you'll end up way ahead of the majority of dieters who, no matter how much they have lost, regain most of it over that same time period.

Points to Remember from This Chapter:

1. After the quick weight loss due to glycogen loss ends, dieters often believe they are stalled when they are actually still losing fat at a slow, normal rate.

2. If your weight loss is really stalled, use a food scale and food software to check that you are really eating the number of grams of carbohydrate you think you're eating.

3. Excess protein can also stall dieters.

4. Excess calories are a major reason for stalls, especially after people have been dieting for a while. The more you have lost, the less you must eat to keep losing.

5. Focusing only on carbohydrates when you are stalled because you are eating excessive calories is foolish.

6. Medical conditions can cause stalls too, and may require medical intervention.

7. Dieters who lose a lot of weight may find that their metabolisms slow dramatically and that maintaining a very large weight loss is extremely difficult. Sometimes it is wisest to end a diet before goal if you have stalled out at the point where cutting any more food out of your diet would make maintenance feel like permanent starvation.

Chapter 14

Maintaining Your Weight Loss

Weight loss is tough. Maintaining that weight loss is tougher. But there are many people out there maintaining long-term low carb weight losses, and there's no reason you can't become one of them.

Research Quantifies How Hard Maintenance Really Is

There are no research studies that track the success of dieters' who have remained on a low carb diet for longer than two years. And even the studies we looked at earlier that tracked low carb dieters for two or three years only gave us averages to tell us how groups of dieters fared as a whole. They didn't tell us how many supposedly low carb dieters were still eating a low carb diet at the end of the two years, nor did they tell us anything about whether the people who stuck to their diets throughout the whole study were able to maintain their weight loss in subsequent years. Chances are that if there had been good news about any of these issues the researchers would have published it, because good long-term results are almost nonexistent in the world of diet research.

The main thing the research tells us is that a very high percentage of low carb dieters dropped out during all the diet studies, many long before a single year was over. So anyone who does manage to stick to their diet for more than a year or two is part of a small, select, and very special group.

The good news is that such people exist. I know quite a few personally, since many are active online. I've met several of them in person over the years, too, and confirmed that they are as slim and fit as they said they were. And, I'm one, too, having maintained a loss of 17% of my starting weight since 2003.

Though we don't have studies about people maintaining weight losses achieved on low carb diets, there *are* studies that track the long-term outcomes of dieters who ate other kinds of diets, and they do have some useful things to teach us.

One study is an analysis that pooled data from 29 smaller studies of dieters who had lost weight in a structured weight-loss program—i.e. a plan like Weight Watchers. It found that once-obese dieters who had lost on average 23% of their starting weight were only able to maintain a weight loss of 3.2% of their starting weight over 5 years. Those who had eaten very low calorie diets regained at a similar rate as those who had not. But because the very low calorie dieters had lost more weight during the initial diet phase they weighed less at the end of the five years, relative to their starting weights. (Anderson, 2001)

The "Look AHEAD" study of 5,145 people with Type 2 diabetes found that people with diabetes did slightly better than the general public at maintaining their weight losses. On average, these dieters with Type 2 diabetes maintained a loss of 4.7% of their starting weight for four years *if* they were given intensive education and hands-on help in doing the initial diet. This help included not only giving dieters specific meal plans but even supplying prepared meals early on in the diet.

These diets were, of course, the high carbohydrate, low fat, low ca-lorie diets doctors recommend for people with diabetes—diets that often ratchet up their hunger. Dieters in this study who were using insulin when they started their diets maintained a fraction of a pound less than those who weren't, but even so, they still did better at main-taining their small average weight loss than did the dieters without diabetes in the Anderson study.

And some of the diabetic dieters given extensive support did *much* better. In the group that received extensive education and support, 23% kept off a loss of more than 10% of their starting weight for four years, and 9% kept off a loss of more than 15%. Though at the other extreme, 4 years after the start of their diets, another 26% of these edu-cated dieters ended up weighing *more* than they did at the start of their diets, and of these 8% ended up 5% heavier than they'd been when they started out.

Dieters with diabetes who were only given vague advice about how to diet and told to consult their doctors if they needed more help did much more poorly than those given extensive support. On average they maintained a weight loss of only 1.1% of their starting weight, but 45% of them ended up heavier than they started out, and of those, 18% had regained 5% more than their starting weight.

This points out how important it is to educate yourself about your diet and to learn the facts about the foods you eat. It also points out how helpful support is. Many of us online find that interacting with supportive people who understand what we're doing helps us stay on track. (Wadden, 2011)

More interesting are the few studies that tease out the behaviors that characterize the dieters who avoid weight gain. As it turns out, these factors are the same ones that were reported in the polls I conducted of successful dieters who had cut down on carbs either to control their blood sugars or lose weight.

Accountability

The single most effective thing people can do to keep from regaining weight is to weigh themselves on a regular basis and go back on their diets as soon as they see any hint of real weight gain. This has long been a common thread in discussions online, but there is also a well-conducted study that backs up this conclusion.

That study followed 318 dieters for 18 months. Over the two years before the study began, these dieters had lost about 20% of their starting weight using a variety of diet strategies. The study broke these dieters into three groups, which were given either face-to-face support, internet chat-group support, or no support.

"Support" in this study meant having the dieters report their weight each week to someone working for the researchers. After they reported their weight, they were given feedback based on whether they had maintained, gained 3-5 lbs, or gained more than 5 pounds. The dieters who reported less than a 3 lbs weekly weight gain—which is well within the normal range of fluctuation due to the weight of food, water weight, and salt intake—were given a trivial reward. Those who gained 3-5 pounds were given "yellow light" status and urged to cut back on their calories. Dieters who had gained more than 5 pounds were assigned "red light" status and told to go back on the diets they had eaten to lose weight.

This support greatly improved the percentage of dieters who did not gain 5 lbs over the 18 month period of the study. The researchers also found that face-to-face support was more effective than chat group support. But this study also found that in all groups, including those getting no support, the dieters who weighed themselves daily were *much* more likely to avoid that 5 lb weight gain. (Wing, 2006)

If you cast your mind back to how hard it was to lose the last pound you lost on your diet, you can see why it is essential to stop any weight regain as soon as starts. Five pounds may not be difficult to lose when you start out on a new diet. But when you are at your diet goal, losing a pound can take weeks, and losing ten may take more months—and more self-restraint—than most long-term dieters have left by the time they reach their goals.

That's why it is so important to take immediate action as soon as you see any hint that your weight is creeping up. That way you can undo any damage with only a few weeks of careful eating. Don't wait until you've gained so much it will take months of stringent dieting that will be exactly like the last months of your diet—when your weight loss had slowed to a crawl.

How true this is was illustrated by what a successful long-term low carb dieter who responded to one of my polls said when asked about whether she had regained any weight. She replied, "The most I've gained above my goal weight is 13 pounds. As soon as I realized what had happened, I cracked down and lost 5 of those pounds in about a week. [This is largely glycogen-related weight loss] I've since gone down another 3-4 pounds a couple of times but I seem to be stuck now at about 8 pounds over goal weight."

Another reported a similar experience saying, "I also weigh myself every day. I think it's important to know where I stand. I would hate to be surprised after a week to find that I'd gained a few pounds. If I'd seen it start to go up a few days earlier, I could have done something about it sooner."

She then added, "I've tried to keep my maintenance weight range to no more than 5 pounds above my goal weight. I've never had a problem sticking to that rule until about a year or so ago. I foolishly thought that I could get away with indulging in high carb goodies while on vacation and managed to gain 8 pounds. I've been struggling ever since then to get my weight back down. Right now I am still about 8 pounds above goal."

Another agreed, saying, "I've just put on 2-3 lbs and will cut out those extra carbs ASAP! I don't wait till I've put on 5 lbs. That's way too much for me to handle."

Some women did report that they don't weigh themselves the week of their periods as they often gain a lot of weight at that time and find it demoralizing.

Other Forms of Accountability

Some successful maintainers not only weigh themselves but every now and then go back to tracking what they are eating with food logs or software. As one of these people explained, "I realized that a tablespoon of double cream was OK, but half the tub wasn't. Any time that my weight starts to creep up, I go back to recording all my food for a while. Just the act of keeping track seems to help."

Of the two groups I have polled, the people with diabetes who eat low carb diets to control their blood sugar seem to do best at long-term maintenance, perhaps because the stakes are so much higher for them. But it may also be because they monitor their blood sugars after meals with their meters, which makes it easier for them to detect when they are going off their food plans.

Many of these dieters with diabetes report that they still eat no more than 30 grams a day of carbohydrate even while in maintenance. Those who eat more—and some do report eating up to 125 grams a day— report that testing their blood sugar after meals is essential. As one of these said, "I continue to test often, because I'm slightly compulsive that way, and because I eat in restaurants a fair amount and it lets me check out new dishes every now and then, and because it keeps me honest."

Others make themselves test their blood sugar after they've eaten something they know isn't good for them, because seeing a high number on the meter reminds them of what's at stake. My own rule for many years has been that I can eat any food I want—as long as I test after eating it.

Seeing ugly numbers on the meter impels some to take immediate corrective action. As one said, "If I test after dinner and it's too high for me, I get on an old exercise bike someone gave me and ride for 20 minutes. That will usually take the numbers down quickly."

In contrast, some weight loss dieters who post on online discussion groups say that they find weighing and testing too confrontational and rely only on how tight their pants feel to monitor whether they have lost weight. But pants stretch out, so you can't rely on sizes to tell you how big you are. Today's size 10 was a size 16, 20 years ago, and stores know you are more likely to buy something if you fit into a smaller size, so they often vanity-size their offerings. Relying on clothing to tell you if you are gaining can result in some nasty surprises.

Low carb discussion boards are full of posts from people who'd been avoiding the scale and wail that they've just came back from a doctor's appointment where they learned they had gained 10 or 15 pounds when they had thought they were maintaining.

One successful maintainer with diabetes tackles the problem of how to deal with the anxiety we feel when a reading is too high with advice that could apply just as well to people who feel anxiety when approaching the scale. "Don't stress over one (or a few) odd high readings. So many things can affect your blood sugar levels [or weight] that it can be hard to pinpoint the cause. Watch for longer-term trends, and then see if you can suss out whatever issue needs to be addressed. Don't beat yourself up over a lapse—just get back on that wagon and keep plugging."

My own experience, and that of quite a few others, is that if we find ourselves avoiding the scale—or the blood sugar meter—it's almost always a sign that we *know* we are eating things that we shouldn't be. If you notice yourself doing that, don't agonize, just get on the scale or get out your meter, assess the damage, and go back onto whatever diet works for you.

Dieters who maintain at a carbohydrate intake level very close to the level where their glycogen starts refilling may find that their weight fluctuates in a way that makes maintenance very frustrating. For me that level was about 70 grams a day. Gaining and losing 3 lbs every few days when maintaining at that level was intolerable, especially since losing glycogen would make me spend way too much time in the bathroom dumping water. I ended up raising my carbs another 10 grams which let me stabilize at the higher weight. Once I got used to carrying a normal load of glycogen I no longer felt bloated the way we do right after glycogen weight comes back on.

The key thing to remember is that accountability requires action. To make maintenance work we have to define some rules ahead of time that tell us what numbers are the numbers where we will take immediate action and what that action will be. It's up to you to decide what those numbers will be and what diet strategy you will use to address them. Just remember, stepping on the scale and wincing at what you see won't keep your weight down, taking steps that very day to cut back on what you're eating will.

Eating Breakfast

A survey of the dieters who reported their habits to the National Weight Control Registry turns up another behavior that seems to be associated with maintaining a significant weight loss for five years or more: eating breakfast. (Wing, 2005)

Protein breakfasts are particularly good at keeping you from getting hungry later on. If you don't eat breakfast because you don't feel hungry first thing in the morning, you may end up doing what a lot of people do when they attempt to lose weight. They eat no breakfast and a very small lunch, thinking this will cut down on their daily food intake. But all it really does is make them so hungry later on that they eat a huge dinner and snack throughout the rest of the evening. Those nighttime snacks can pack on a lot of extra pounds. If you start your day with a high protein breakfast that damps down hunger, you are less likely to end up hungry as the day goes on, and that will make it easier to avoid that evening snacking.

The other thing eating breakfast does is to knock down your fasting blood sugars, which can be higher than any other reading you would see during the rest of the day. Blood sugars may rise a bit, first thing in the morning, even in people who eat low carb diets. This is due to something called "Dawn effect." It's a normal reaction to the hormones our bodies secrete right before we wake up, whose purpose is to raise our blood sugar to give us extra energy to go out and hunt the food we'll need to start the day. In some people this dawn effect can be quite strong, and though their blood sugars are normal for the rest of the day, they may be pre-diabetic or even diabetic first thing in the morning. Eating breakfast will almost always knock these higher than normal levels right back down to normal.

Exercise

The same nutritionists who insist that the only way to lose weight is to eat a low fat diet also argue that exercise is essential to maintaining weight loss. There are plenty of studies that suggest that people who exercise maintain slightly more weight loss than those who don't. But the actual difference between those who do and don't exercise is not great.

One study quantified this for a group of premenopausal women followed for 6 years after they achieved a significant weight loss. In this group, 80% of the women regained more than 30% of their intentional weight loss. The researchers found that in the group as a whole, those who exercised for 30 minutes a day regained an average of 3 lbs less than those who didn't. When women who were still overweight at the end of their diets exercised, they regained an average of 5 lbs less than those who didn't. However, this study did not report the weight losses and gains as a percentage of these women's starting weight, which would have been a more revealing statistic and might have made it clear if these slight differences in how much they regained had anything to do with how much the women had originally lost.

In this particular study, the researchers found that jogging and running were associated with the least regain, but both those kinds of exercise are very hard on the knees. So for those of us who want to ensure life-long fitness, those forms of exercise may be less healthy over long term than more moderate exercises that don't result in the knee replacement surgeries that severely curtail our ability to exercise as we age. (Mekary, 2010)

Another attempt to quantify the impact of exercise in women's weight maintenance concluded that while exercise made no difference during the weight loss phase of their diets, women who exercised for 4.6 hours a week were more likely to maintain a 10% weight loss—*but only if they also restricted their caloric intake.* (Jakicic, 2008)

The problem with these studies, however, is that the data about how much exercise people do is usually gathered by asking them, and this may lead people to exaggerate. It's likely many people reported the amount of exercise they wish they did, rather than what they actually do. Who, after all, is going to tell a doctor or other authority figure, "I never do anything but sit around playing on my computer, and the only exercise I get is from laughing when I watch cat videos on You-Tube?"

That this might have been the case in the Mekary study reported above is suggested by the fact that these women also self-reported an intake of only 3 grams a day of trans fat, even though the study was conducted in 1991, when there was transfat in all margarines and most packaged foods.

The other problem with the studies that promote the helpfulness of exercise is that even the dieters who exercise still regain so much of the weight they lost. Since many of these women were still quite over-weight at the end of their diets, the 3 or 4 pounds they kept off through exercise palls in the face of the 20 to 50 lbs they put back on.

In two separate polls I've run where I've asked people who have maintained a low carb weight loss for three years or more how impor-tant they found exercise, half of those who replied in each survey said that exercise made no difference in their ability to maintain.

This has been my own experience, too. Going to the gym gives me nicer muscles and better cardiac capacity, but it doesn't make any dif-ference in my weight or my blood sugar control.

This was echoed by statements made by several successful main-tainers who responded to my polls. One said, "I exercise for my men-tal health and muscle definition, not for weight loss." Another ex-plained, "I don't find exercise to be at all important in regard to weight loss or maintenance. I did no exercise at all during my 50 pound weight loss. I'm not keen on much physical activity, and I'm never going to be a professional athlete, so any amount of exercise that I do is never going to be enough to affect my weight one way or the other. However, I do try to do an hour of Callanetics twice a week, because it makes me feel good, and it improves the way my body looks."

Another successful maintainer says, "I've never noticed any effect on weight loss or maintenance. Exercise helps my mood, energy, strength, and lower back problems." Yet another adds, "Exercise makes me feel less flabby and lazy. I also use it for mental clarity and bone strength for my future years. I don't base my food intake on my exercise output."

This is an important point, because it is very easy to gain weight if you believe you've burned as many calories during your workout as you saw displayed on the machines at the gym. This was discussed in an article published in the New York Times that was titled "Putting Very Little Weight in Calorie Counting Methods." (Kolata, 2007)

The author of the article, pointed out that any two individuals will vary greatly in how many calories they burn while doing the same amount of exercise, even if they maintain the same percentage of total heart rate capacity, so the readouts on the gym equipment are highly misleading. Age and weight, which are all the machines ask about, are only a few of the many factors that determine how many calories you are actually burning. Your height, your muscle mass, your gender, and the genetics that determine how well your mitochondria burn fuel also factor in.

Something called the "training effect" also decreases how much you burn, because the *more* you do a certain activity, the *fewer* calories you burn each time you do it. Kolata quotes a researcher saying, "Subjects rode stationary bicycles six days a week for 12 weeks. They ended up burning 10% fewer calories at a given level of effort after their training."

Among those with diabetes who I've polled, half also report that they don't find exercise essential or even useful for maintaining. In fact, some of those who reported regaining significant amounts of weight after reaching goal are among those who exercised most faithfully, which makes you wonder if exercising makes people give themselves permission to eat more than they otherwise would.

One reason that these people with diabetes didn't focus on exercise is that cutting way down on their carbohydrate intake had been enough to give them the extremely good blood sugar control which was their primary objective. As one successful diabetic maintainer explained, "It is good for my general health. However, whether walking 5 miles as fast as I can in nice weather, or getting almost no exercise at all when snowed in. in the winter, my glucose control is the same— exceptional."

The group of people with diabetes I polled tends to be older than the weight loss dieters I met through online low carb support forums. Many are coping with physical conditions that severely limit their mobility. After a cancer diagnosis, surgery, and chemo one woman said, "I love my exercise, but as I do less not much has changed." Another says, "Exercise is irrelevant to me (well, to my control). I have other medical issues which sometimes limit the kinds of exercise I can do. While exercise is obviously beneficial to general health, I don't want my diabetes control to be dependent on a level of exercise I might not be able to maintain."

One of these successful maintainers told me, "I don't exercise at all because of physical disabilities (I use a power chair and a motorized mobility scooter)." Even so he has been able to maintain a weight loss of 45 lbs and keep his blood sugar in a healthy range.

Half of both groups I polled *did* report that they found exercise useful in maintaining their weight loss. And some of the people with Type 2 diabetes also reported that exercise helps them lower their blood sugar, like the one who wrote, "My perception is that it helps with BGs [blood glucose] — but that good, vigorous walking is more effective than other forms of exercise. If I take a two- or three-mile walk at a good clip, my BGs really benefit for a couple of days. I don't know that exercise has any effect on my weight, but it does help keep me fit."

The bottom line seems to be that whatever the benefits of regular exercise, and there undoubtedly are many, it isn't required for the maintenance of either a significant weight loss or better blood sugars. Knowing this should be comforting to people who can't indulge in vigorous exercise and reassure them that with a low carb eating strategy that keeps their blood sugar completely normal they can control their weight while doing only the amount of physical activity they are capable of.

How Much Carb Can You Add When You Get To Goal?

One question many low carb dieters have when they reach their weight goal is how much carbohydrate can they add back into their diet. The answer to this question depends entirely on how your blood sugar responds as you raise your carbohydrate intake.

Adding carbs quickly can provoke the same sudden glycogen-related weight gain and hunger attacks that happen when people crash off their diets. So the best way to raise your carbohydrate intake is very slowly, adding only 5 to 10 grams at a time.

The best way to learn exactly how many grams of carbs you can add is to repeat the steps we described in the section on "How to test your blood sugar." Before you start adding back carbs, test your blood sugar 1 and 2 hours after a normal meal. Then add 5 to 10 grams to your next meal and test again.

Remember that if you have been eating a ketogenic diet it will take up to three days for your enzymes to upregulate so that you can burn glucose efficiently again. If you see a sudden spike after raising carbs, accompanied by weight gain that suggests you have started to put on glycogen, keep eating at that carb level, wait three days, and test again.

Any time you see your blood sugar going over 140 mg/dl, you've pushed your blood sugar into the unhealthy range and need to back off the carbs. If you don't go over 120 mg/dl, you're fine. If you are still feeling hungrier than usual after you have spent a week at your new higher carb level and have given your body time to adapt, you may need to cut back, too. Hunger is always a sign that you are eating more carbs that your body is comfortable with.

Raising carbs this way sounds good in theory, but in practice many dieters who have been on ketogenic diets for a long time go overboard when they add back carbs. This is especially likely to happen to dieters who have been very rigid while losing weight and have let themselves build up a backlog of frustrated food desires. This is one reason why it's a good idea to design your diet so that, even if it produces a slower weight loss, it prevents you from building up the kind of deferred cravings that can make maintenance difficult.

My poll of people who were successful in using a low carb diet for weight loss, as opposed to blood sugar control, found that, while a few of them have remained at a ketogenic level for many years after reaching goal, most of them have raised their carbs. When asked by how much, several explained that their intake fluctuates from day to day and even from meal to meal.

Several say they have days when they eat between 100 and 130 grams of carbs, but that they also have other days when their carb intake is much lower. As one person explains, "If I have a higher-carb breakfast, I compensate for it by eating lower-carb items the rest of the day. If I have a higher-carb dinner, I'll compensate the next day a bit." Quite a few people gave their daily carb input as fluctuating from "40 to 100 grams."

When they describe what kinds of carbs they've added back into their daily diet, these successful dieters report that they've added more fruits, potatoes, and breads like sourdough or quality whole grain breads made with visible kernels of grain. Some have added back in the starchier colorful vegetables like winter squash and sweet potatoes, foods which are rich in nutrients.

As one explains, "A big thing I pay attention to is not to eat too many carbs at any one meal to be sure my blood sugar doesn't go way up." Portion control can really help here. Pile a sandwich's worth of filling on one slice of bread cut in half, rather than two. Eat half a small baked red potato, rather than a whole large Idaho.

Quite a few people mention that sugar gets them in trouble. As one woman explains, "For me, the only thing that works is abstinence when it comes to sugar. One bite and it's down hill from there. "

Raising Carbs When You Have Abnormal Blood Sugars

The picture is much different for those I polled who are eating low carb diets to control abnormal blood sugars. Though several of them reported eating between 100 and 130 grams a day, the majority were still eating at ketogenic levels. For some this was because they enjoy the food and feel better eating at that level. For others, the reason they stayed at so low a carb intake level was because they couldn't find a doctor who would prescribe the medications that would keep their blood sugars in control if they were to eat more carbs.

The diet does such a good job of controlling blood sugars that when many people with prediabetes or diabetes go to a doctor for help, they come away empty-handed. The doctors take one look at their blood work and declare that they don't have diabetes and therefore don't need treatment. Some of the successful low carb dieters with diabetes I polled remarked on this.

One said, "I wish I could find a doctor who wouldn't blow me off when I say that I want to be on some sort of insulin regimen, so I don't totally burn out my pancreas, but no luck so far with that." Another adds, "My PCP doesn't think that, with an A1C of less than 6.0, I have any blood sugar control issues."

Extending Your Diet Success to the Rest of Your Life

The fact that people with diabetes maintain better on all kinds of low carb diets and do a better job of sticking to ketogenic diets long-term points to one essential point that can help you succeed at maintaining your own diet achievements for life.

People with diabetes do a better job at maintaining because they know exactly *why* they must cut the carbs and when they cut those carbs, they get exactly the result they hoped for: the normal blood sugars that mean they won't have to suffer the blindness, kidney failure, amputation and death that so many of them have seen devastate their relatives. Because the diet does what they need it to do, they remain motivated.

For people who diet for weight loss, achieving their weight loss goal can make it harder to stay motivated. Not only do they lose the daily motivation of seeing the number on the scale go down, but the end of the diet forces them to confront any unrealistic hopes and dreams that may have fueled their weight loss journeys.

Because so many low carb diets end before the dieters get to their goals, they may come away feeling they don't have what it takes to succeed—even though, by any objective measure, these people have lost far more weight than the average dieter.

But even those who do reach their diet goals may experience a painful letdown when they have to face the fact that no matter how much they now weigh, they are still the same person, with the same family, the same employment situation, and the same friends. If they have secretly been hoping that a new body shape would give them a more fulfilling life, the end of the diet may confront them with how far they still are from the life they dreamed of living.

A brilliant book published back in 1985 called *Keeping It off: Winning at Weight Loss* reported on a group of people who had lost 20% or more of their body weight and kept it off for five years or more. The authors found that these successful dieters shared one highly relevant trait, which was that their diets were only a *part* of what these people changed about their lives.

Many of the women who succeeded in dieting also took steps to change the other aspects of their lives that had caused them to feel hopeless, such as bad marriages or career dead ends. Their diet success taught them that they could take control of their own lives and, having learned that, they moved on to make other important changes.

So if you find yourself having a hard time maintaining your weight loss, or feel depressed in the months after you achieve your goal, take a long hard look at the hopes and dreams you may have thought your weight loss would make possible. If they are still unfulfilled, take the rest of the steps required to make those dreams come true.

You've already shown that you can work hard to make a major improvement in your life by losing weight. This is something many people never manage to do. Pause to appreciate what you've done. Applaud yourself for your accomplishment. Then draw on the same dedication, ability to learn, and willingness to work that you put into your weight loss to make the *rest* of your life as good as it can be.

Points to Remember from This Chapter:

1. Maintenance is tough and few dieters maintain their weight losses very well over time.

2. Accountability is the key: weighing frequently and taking immediate steps to lose the first pounds that come back on will lead to long-term success.

3. Eating breakfast is a characteristic of successful maintainers.

4. Half of dieters find that exercise makes no difference in their ability to maintain, whatever other effects it has. Research suggests that exercise helps people keep off only a few more pounds. At the same time, exercising may tempt people to eat more than they otherwise would, because people overestimate how many calories exercise burns.

5. How much additional carbohydrate you can eat at the end of your diet depends on how well your blood sugars function.

6. Use the dedication you put into achieving your successful weight loss to tackle the other issues in your life you need to change to be truly happy.

Acknowledgments

Dr. Richard K. Bernstein gave me the basic understanding I needed to get started studying blood sugar. His book, *Dr. Bernstein's Diabetes Solution*, also taught me that the levels most doctors consider normal aren't. It's essential reading for anyone with diabetes or prediabetes.

I'm also grateful to the hundreds of people who posted on the alt.support.diet.low-carb newsgroup in those glorious days before it was overwhelmed by spam. They taught me a lot about successful dieting and about the psychology of dieters. Without their many practical suggestions I doubt I'd have been able to stay on a ketogenic diet as long as I did. Special thanks to a.s.d.l-c's Carol Ann. for running the monthly challenges and to Lyle McDonald for inspiring me to delve into the published research.

My greatest breakthroughs in understanding the low carb diet came from reading the posts on alt.support.diabetes. It was there I first read Jennifer's brilliant advice to newbies, the "test, test, test" advice I've been popularizing for a decade. It's unsurpassed as a simple but totally effective way to control blood sugar. The denizens of the diabetes newsgroup taught me that it wasn't always necessary to eat a ketogenic diet to control blood sugar. They also made me aware of how greatly people vary in their ability to tolerate carbs.

My thanks go out to everyone who replied to the polls I posted over the years on my blog and various online discussion forums. Your answers gave me insight into the wide range of strategies people use to keep their blood sugars normal and their weight in check.

Jimmy Moore gets credit for getting me to sit down and write this book. He asked great questions when he interviewed me that started me thinking. He was also kind enough to review an early version of this manuscript. His enthusiastic response gave me the confidence to keep working on it.

Peter Atwood took time out of his very busy schedule to give my manuscript a thorough copyedit. He challenged me to back up everything I'd said and brought up several important points that helped me make the book much better. Alicia Rasley, editor extraordinaire, also contributed valuable insights.

Dr. Stephan Guyenet, author of the extremely informative "Whole Health Source" blog, was extremely generous with his time and willingness to review and comment on the science discussed in these pages. Though he didn't always agree with points I've raised, he was open to considering that future research might validate some of them. His input made this book much better. Any scientific errors remaining in the text are entirely mine.

References

A.D.A.M. Medical Encyclopedia: Metabolic acidosis
http://www.ncbi.nlm.nih.gov/pubmedhealth/PMH0001376/

Acheson K J et al: Glycogen synthesis versus lipogenesis after a 500 gram carbohydrate meal in man. *Metabolism*. Volume 31, Issue 12, December 1982, Pages 1234-1240
http://www.sciencedirect.com/science/article/pii/0026049582900105

ADA: Diagnosis and Classification of Diabetes Mellitus. *Diabetes Care*. January 2010 vol. 33 no. Supplement 1 S62-S69 http://care.diabetesjournals.org/content/33/Supplement_1/S62.full

Ahmadi SA, et al: The impact of low serum triglyceride on LDL-cholesterol estimation. *Arch Iran Med*. 2008 May; 11(3):318-21 http://www.ncbi.nlm.nih.gov/pubmed/18426324

Althuis MD et al: Glucose and insulin responses to dietary chromium supplements: a meta-analysis. *Am J Clin Nutr*. 2002 Jul; 76(1):148-55 http://www.ajcn.org/content/76/1/148.abstract

An epidemic of obesity myths. http://www.obesitymyths.com/myth2.2.htm

Anderson JW et al: Long-term weight-loss maintenance: a meta-analysis of US studies. *Am J Clin Nutr*. 2001; 74:579-84 http://www.indiana.edu/~k662/articles/obesity/wt%20main%20Anderson%202001.pdf

Anderson, RA: Chromium, Glucose Intolerance and Diabetes. *Journal of the American College of Nutrition*. Vol. 17, No. 6, 548-555 (1998) http://www.jacn.org/content/17/6/548.full

Audette R et al: *NeanderThin: Eat Like a Caveman to Achieve a Lean, Strong, Healthy Body*. St. Martins Paperbacks, New York, 2000. ISBN 978-0312975913

Austin GL, et al: A very low-carbohydrate diet improves gastroesophageal reflux and its symptoms. *Dig Dis Sci*. 2006 Aug; 51(8):1307-12. Epub 2006 Jul 27.
http://www.ncbi.nlm.nih.gov/pubmed/16871438?dopt=Abstract

Bank IM et al: Sudden cardiac death in association with the ketogenic diet. *Pediatr Neurol*. 2008 Dec; 39(6):429-31. http://www.ncbi.nlm.nih.gov/pubmed/19027591

Bardini G et al: Inflammation markers and metabolic characteristics of subjects with one-hour plasma glucose levels. *Diabetes Care* Published online before print November 16, 2009.
http://care.diabetesjournals.org/content/early/2009/11/12/dc09-1342.abstract

Bariatric Surgery Source: Gastric Bypass Surgery Deaths: 3 Most Common Causes & Other Risks of Gastric Bypass. http://www.bariatric-surgery-source.com/gastric-bypass-surgery-deaths.html

Batterham RL: Inhibition of food intake in obese subjects by peptide YY3-36. *The New England Journal of Medicine*. (Sept 2003) 349 (10): 941-8. doi:10.1056/NEJMoa030204. PMID 12954742
http://www.nejm.org/doi/full/10.1056/NEJMoa030204

Berenson A: Disparity Emerges in Lilly Data on Schizophrenia Drug. *New York Times*. Dec 26, 2006
http://www.nytimes.com/2006/12/21/business/21drug.html?scp=1&sq=December%2021,%202006%20Zyprexa&st=cse

Bergstrom et al: Diet, muscle glycogen and physical performance. *Acta Physiol Scand*. 1967; 71:140-50

Berkeley Wellness Letter, February 2004. Iron. http://www.wellnessletter.com/html/ds/dsIron.php

Bernstein RK: *Doctor Bernstein's Diabetes Solution*, 3nd ed. Little Brown & Co, NY, 2007 ISBN 978-0-316-16716-1

Bhutani S et al: Improvements in Coronary Heart Disease Risk Indicators by Alternate-Day Fasting Involve Adipose Tissue Modulations. *Obesity*. (2010)
http://www.nature.com/oby/journal/vaop/ncurrent/full/oby201054a.html

Bjelakovic G et al: Mortality in randomized trials of antioxidant supplements for primary and secondary prevention: systematic review and meta-analysis. *JAMA*. 2007 Feb 28; 297(8):842-57
http://www.ncbi.nlm.nih.gov/pubmed/17327526?dopt=Abstract

Blevins SM et al: Effect of Cinnamon on Glucose and Lipid Levels in Non-Insulin-Dependent Type 2 Diabetes. *Diabetes Care*. September 2007 vol. 30 no. 9 2236-2237
http://care.diabetesjournals.org/content/30/9/2236.full

Blood Sugar 101: A1c and Post-Meal Blood Sugars Predict Heart Attack.
http://www.bloodsugar101.com/15945839.php

Blood Sugar 101: Causes. http://www.phlaunt.com/diabetes/14046739.php

Blood Sugar 101: Diabetic Tendon Problems. http://www.bloodsugar101.com/16162241.php

Blood Sugar 101: Drugs that Force the Pancreas to Produce (or Over-produce) Insulin
http://www.bloodsugar101.com/25311847.php

Blood Sugar 101: Misdiagnosis By Design - The Story Behind the ADA Diagnostic Criteria,
http://www.phlaunt.com/diabetes/14046782.php

Blood Sugar 101: More insight into why A1c doesn't match your meter measurements.
http://diabetesupdate.blogspot.com/2008/03/more-insight-into-why-a1c-doesnt-match.html

Blood Sugar 101: No, weight loss surgery does not cure diabetes.
http://diabetesupdate.blogspot.com/2012/03/no-wls-does-not-cure-diabetes-study-by.html

Blood Sugar 101: Research Connecting Organ Damage with Blood Sugar Level.
http://www.bloodsugar101.com/14045678.php

Blood Sugar 101:http://diabetesupdate.blogspot.com/2011/12/mitochondrial-diabetes-another-non.html

Boden G et al: Effect of a Low-Carbohydrate Diet on Appetite, Blood Glucose Levels, and Insulin Resistance
in Obese Patients with Type 2 Diabetes. *Annals of Internal Medicine.* March 15, 2005, vol. 142 no. 6
403-411 http://www.annals.org/content/142/6/403.full.pdf+html

Bolland MJ et al: Vascular events in healthy older women receiving calcium supplementation: randomised
controlled trial *BMJ.* 2008 February 2; 336(7638): 262-266.
http://www.ncbi.nlm.nih.gov/pmc/articles/PMC2222999/

Brinkworth GD et al: Long-term Effects of a Very Low-Carbohydrate Diet and a Low-Fat Diet on Mood and
Cognitive Function. *Arch Intern Med.* 2009; 169(20):1873-1880 http://archinte.ama-
assn.org/cgi/content/full/169/20/1873

Brinkworth GD et al: Long-term effects of a very-low-carbohydrate weight loss diet compared with an isocaloric low-fat diet after 12 mo. *Am J Clin Nutr.* July 2009 vol. 90 no. 1 23-32 doi:
10.3945/ajcn.2008.27326 http://www.ajcn.org/content/90/1/23.full

Brown AM: Astrocyte glycogen and brain energy metabolism. *Glia.* 2007 Sep;55(12):1263-71
http://www.ncbi.nlm.nih.gov/pubmed/17659525

Browning J D et al: Alterations in hepatic glucose and energy metabolism as a result of calorie and carbohydrate restriction. *Hepatology.* Volume 48, Issue 5, pages 1487-1496, November 2008

Butler, AE: ß-Cell Deficit and Increased ß-Cell Apoptosis in Humans With Type 2 Diabetes. *Diabetes.* January
2003 vol. 52 no. 1 102-110 http://diabetes.diabetesjournals.org/content/52/1/102.full

Campbell B: Glycemic Load Vs. Glycemic Index. (undated) http://www.nsca-
lift.org/HotTopic/download/Glycemic%20Load.pdf

Canavan B et al: Effects of Physiological Leptin Administration on Markers of Inflammation, Platelet Activa-
tion, and Platelet Aggregation during Caloric Deprivation. *The Journal of Clinical Endocrinology &
Metabolism.* Vol. 90, No. 10, 2005, 5779-5785 http://jcem.endojournals.org/content/90/10/5779.full

Carillo S et al: The effects of a low-carbohydrate versus low-fat diet on adipocytokines in severely obese
adults: three-year follow-up of a randomized trial. *European Review for Medical and Pharmacologi-
cal Sciences.* 2006; 10: 99-106 http://www.europeanreview.org/pdf/375.pdf

Carwile JL et al: Canned Soup Consumption and Urinary Bisphenol A: A Randomized Crossover Trial. *JAMA.*
2011; 306(20):2218-2220. doi: 10.1001/jama.2011.1721 http://jama.ama-
assn.org/content/306/20/2218.2.short

Castelli WP: Lipids, risk factors and ischaemic heart disease. Framingham Cardiovascular Institute, *Atherosclerosis.* 1996 Jul; 124 Suppl:S1-9. http://www.ncbi.nlm.nih.gov/pubmed/8831910

CDC: Number of Americans with Diabetes Rises to Nearly 26 Million
http://www.cdc.gov/media/releases/2011/p0126_diabetes.html

Center SA et al: Clinical and Metabolic Effects of Rapid Weight Loss in Obese Pet Cats and the Influence of
Supplemental Oral L-Carnitine. *Journal of Veterinary Internal Medicine.* Volume 14, Issue 6, pages
598-608, November 2000 http://onlinelibrary.wiley.com/doi/10.1111/j.1939-
1676.2000.tb02283.x/abstract

Chan HL: How Should We Manage Patients With Non-alcoholic Fatty Liver Disease in 2007? J *Gastroenterol
Hepatol.* 2007;22(6):801-808. http://www.medscape.com/viewarticle/559337

Christensen JS: What is Normal Glucose? - Continuous Glucose Monitoring Data from Healthy Subjects. On
the occasion of the Annual Meeting of the EASD, Copenhagen, 13-Sep-06 http://www.diabetes-
symposium.org/index.php?menu=view&chart=4&id=322

Codru N et al: Diabetes in Relation to Serum Levels of Polychlorinated Biphenyls and Chlorinated Pesticides in
Adult Native Americans. *Environ Health Perspect.* 2007 October; 115(10): 1442-1447.doi:
10.1289/ehp.10315 http://www.ncbi.nlm.nih.gov/pmc/articles/PMC2022671/

Coleman M et al: Urinary ketones reflect serum ketone concentration but do not relate to weight loss in overweight premenopausal women following a low-carbohydrate/high-protein diet. *Journal of the Ameri-*

can Dietetic Association. Volume 105 , Issue 4 , April 2005 Pages 608 - 611
http://www.journals.elsevierhealth.com/periodicals/yjada/article/S0002-8223(05)00005-2/abstract

Colvin RH et al: *Keeping It Off: Winning At Weight Loss.* Simon & Schuster (October 1985) ISBN 978-0671532949

Consumer Affairs: Kimkins Diet Rolls On Despite Founder's Excess Poundage.
http://www.consumeraffairs.com/news04/2008/02/kimkins.html

Consumer Alert: Hoodia Gordonii weight loss pills scam exposed by independent investigation
http://www.naturalnews.com/006016.html

Cordain L: *The Paleo Diet: Lose Weight and Get Healthy by Eating the Foods You Were Designed to Eat.* Wiley, NY, 2010. Revised. ISBN 978-047091302

Croen LA et al: Antidepressant Use During Pregnancy and Childhood Autism Spectrum Disorders. *Arch Gen Psychiatry.* 2011; 68(11):1104-1112. http://archpsyc.ama-assn.org/cgi/content/short/archgenpsychiatry.2011.73

Culver AL et al: Statin Use and Risk of Diabetes Mellitus in Postmenopausal Women in the Women's Health Initiative. *Arch Intern Med.* 2012; 172(2):144-152. http://archinte.ama-assn.org/cgi/content/abstract/172/2/144

Dansinger ML, et al: Comparison of the Atkins, Ornish, Weight Watchers, and Zone Diets for Weight Loss and Heart Disease Risk Reduction: A Randomized Trial. *JAMA.* 2005; 293(1):43-53. http://jama.ama-assn.org/content/293/1/43.full

de Carvalho PP et al: GLUT4 protein is differently modulated during development of obesity in monosodium glutamate-treated mice. *Life Sci.* 2002 Sep 6; 71(16):1917-28
http://www.ncbi.nlm.nih.gov/pubmed/12175706

de Moraes C. et al: Serum Leptin Level in Hypertensive Middle-Aged Obese Women. *The Endocrinologist.* July/August 2005 - Volume 15 - Issue 4 - pp 219-221
http://journals.lww.com/theendocrinologist/pages/articleviewer.aspx?year=2005&issue=07000&article=00007&type=abstract

Diabetes in Control: New Alterations Found in Young Adults with Type 2 Diabetes, March 15, 2010
http://www.diabetesincontrol.com/index.php?option=com_content&view=article&id=9073&catid=53&Itemid=8

Diabetes in Control: Gymnema. Effect of Extended Release Gymnema Sylvestre Leaf Extract (Beta Fast GXR)
http://www.diabetesincontrol.com/articles/uncategorized/10355-effect-of-extended-release-gymnema-sylvestre-leaf-extract-beta-fast-gxr

Diabetes Update: Statins make you fat and insulin resistant. http://diabetesupdate.blogspot.com/2008/04/statins-make-you-fat-and-insulin.html

Dubois A: Diet and gastric digestion. *Am J Clin Nutr.* November 1985 vol. 42 no. 5 1003-1005http://www.ajcn.org/content/42/5/1003.full.pdf

Eades M et al: *Protein Power: The High-Protein/Low-Carbohydrate Way to Lose Weight, Feel Fit, and Boost Your Health--in Just Weeks!* Bantam (June 1, 1999) ISBN: 978-0553380781

EPA: Perfluorooctanoic Acid (PFOA) and Fluorinated Telomers http://www.epa.gov/oppt/pfoa

Esposito K et al: Post-Meal Glucose Peaks at Home Associate with Carotid Intima-Media Thickness in Type 2 Diabetes. *The Journal of Clinical Endocrinology & Metabolism* April 1, 2008 vol. 93 no. 4 1345-1350

Essah PA et al: Effect of Macronutrient Composition on Postprandial Peptide YY Levels. *The Journal of Clinical Endocrinology & Metabolism.* 92(10) (2007):4052-4055
http://jcem.endojournals.org/content/92/10/4052.short

Fabbrini E et al: Intrahepatic fat, not visceral fat, is linked with metabolic complications of obesity. Elisa *PNAS.* Published online before print August 24, 2009.
http://www.pnas.org/content/early/2009/08/21/0904944106.abstract explained in Diabetes in Control: Liver Fat Has Greater Impact on Health than Abdominal Fat.
http://www.diabetesincontrol.com/index.php?option=com_content&view=article&id=8301&catid=1&Itemid=17

FDA: Bisphenol A (BPA)
http://www.fda.gov/Food/FoodIngredientsPackaging/ucm166145.htm?utm_source=fdaSearch&utm_medium=website&utm_term=BPA%202012&utm_content=1

Fernández-Real JM et al:Cross-Talk Between Iron Metabolism and Diabetes. Diabetes. August 2002 vol. 51 no. 8 2348-2354 http://diabetes.diabetesjournals.org/content/57/6/1638.abstract

Festa A et al: ß-Cell Dysfunction in Subjects With Impaired Glucose Tolerance and Early Type 2 Diabetes: Comparison of Surrogate Markers With First-Phase Insulin Secretion From an Intravenous Glucose Tolerance Test. *Diabetes.* June 2008 vol. 57 no. 6 1638-1644
http://diabetes.diabetesjournals.org/content/57/6/1638.abstract

Foster GD et al: Weight and Metabolic Outcomes After 2 Years on a Low-Carbohydrate Versus Low-Fat Diet: A Randomized Trial. *Ann Intern Med.* 2010; 153:147-157. http://www.annals.org/content/153/3/147.abstract

Foster-Powell K et al: International table of glycemic index and glycemic load values. *American Journal of Clinical Nutrition.* Vol. 76, No. 1, 5-56, 2002 http://www.ajcn.org/content/76/1/5.full

Foster-Schubert KE et al: Acyl and Total Ghrelin Are Suppressed Strongly by Ingested Proteins, Weakly by Lipids, and Biphasically by Carbohydrates. *The Journal of Clinical Endocrinology & Metabolism.* May 1, 2008 vol. 93 no. 5 1971-1979 http://jcem.endojournals.org/content/93/5/1971.full

Freeman R et al:Assessing Impaired Glucose Tolerance and Insulin Resistance in Polycystic Ovarian Syndrome with a Muffin Test: An Alternative to the Glucose Tolerance Test , *Endocrine Practice.* Volume 16, Number 5 / September-October 2010, Pages810-817 http://www.ncbi.nlm.nih.gov/pubmed/20439247

Futterman LG, Lemberg L. Fifty percent of patients with coronary artery disease do not have any of the conventional risk factors. *Am J Crit Care.* 1998 May; 7(3):240-4 http://www.ncbi.nlm.nih.gov/pubmed/9579251?dopt=Abstract

Gannon MC et al: Effect of a High-Protein, Low-Carbohydrate Diet on Blood Glucose Control in People With Type 2 Diabetes. *Diabetes.* September 2004 vol. 53 no. 9 2375-2382. http://diabetes.diabetesjournals.org/content/53/9/2375.full.pdf

Gardner CD, et al: Comparison of the Atkins, Zone, Ornish, and LEARNWeight Loss Study: Comparison of the Atkins, Zone, Ornish, and LEARN Diets for Change in Weight and Related Risk Factors Among Overweight Premenopausal Women: The A TO Z Weight Loss Study: A Randomized Trial. *JAMA.* 2007; 297(9):969-977 http://jama.ama-assn.org/cgi/content/full/297/9/969

Genaw L: Linda's Low Carb Menus & Recipes http://www.genaw.com/lowcarb/

Gulseth HL et al: Serum Vitamin D Concentration Does Not Predict Insulin Action or Secretion in European Subjects With the Metabolic Syndrome. *Diabetes Care.* April 2010 vol. 33 no. 4 923-925. doi: 10.2337/dc09-1692 http://care.diabetesjournals.org/content/33/4/923.abstract

Guyenet S: Insulin and Obesity http://wholehealthsource.blogspot.com/2012/01/insulin-and-obesity-another-nail-in.html

Guyenet S: Can Vitamin K2 Reverse Arterial Calcification? http://wholehealthsource.blogspot.com/2008/11/can-vitamin-k2-reverse-arterial.html

Halldorsson TI, et al: Prenatal Exposure to Perfluorooctanoate and Risk of Overweight at 20 Years of Age: A Prospective Cohort Study. *Environ Health Perspect.* 2012. http://ehp03.niehs.nih.gov/article/info%3Adoi%2F10.1289%2Fehp.1104034

Halton TL et al: The Effects of High Protein Diets on Thermogenesis, Satiety and Weight Loss: A Critical Review. *J Am Coll Nutr.* October 2004 vol. 23 no. 5 373-385 http://www.jacn.org/content/23/5/373.abstract

Harris ES J et al: Heavy metal and pesticide content in commonly prescribed individual raw Chinese Herbal Medicines. *Science of The Total Environment.* Volume 409, Issue 20, 15 September 2011, Pages 4297-4305 http://www.ncbi.nlm.nih.gov/pubmed/21824641

Harrison SA et al: Orlistat for overweight subjects with nonalcoholic steatohepatitis: A randomized, prospective trial. *Hepatology.* Volume 49, Issue 1, pages 80-86, January 2009 http://onlinelibrary.wiley.com/doi/10.1002/hep.22575/abstract

Harvard Health Publications: Glycemic index and glycemic load for 100+ foods http://www.health.harvard.edu/newsweek/Glycemic_index_and_glycemic_load_for_100_foods.htm

Haukeland JW et al: Metformin in patients with non-alcoholic fatty liver disease: A randomized, controlled trial. *Scandinavian journal of gastroenterology.* 2009, vol. 44, no7, pp. 853-860 http://cat.inist.fr/?aModele=afficheN&cpsidt=21677571

Haye MR et al: A Carbohydrate-Restricted Diet Alters Gut Peptides and Adiposity Signals in Men and Women with Metabolic Syndrome. *J Nutr.* 137: 1944-1950, 2007 http://jn.nutrition.org/content/137/8/1944.short

He K et al: Association of Monosodium Glutamate Intake With Overweight in Chinese Adults: The INTERMAP Study. *Obesity.* (2008) 16 8, 1875-1880. http://www.nature.com/oby/journal/v16/n8/abs/oby2008274a.html

Heller RF et al: *The Carbohydrate Addict's Diet: The Lifelong Solution to Yo-Yo Dieting* Signet, New York, 1993. ISBN 978-0451173393

Higgins JA: Whole Grains, Legumes, and the Subsequent Meal Effect: Implications for Blood Glucose Control and the Role of Fermentation. *Journal of Nutrition and Metabolism.* Volume 2012 (2012), Article ID 829238, 7 pages http://www.hindawi.com/journals/jnume/2012/829238/

Hodgson JM et al: Coenzyme Q10 improves blood pressure and glycaemic control: a controlled trial in subjects with type 2 diabetes. *European Journal of Clinical Nutrition.* (2002) 56, 1137 - 1142 http://www.ncbi.nlm.nih.gov/pubmed/12428181

House AA et al: Effect of B-Vitamin Therapy on Progression of Diabetic Nephropathy: A Randomized Controlled Trial. *JAMA.* 2010; 303(16):1603-1609 http://jama.ama-assn.org/content/303/16/1603.long

Hugo ER et al: Bisphenol A at Environmentally Relevant Doses Inhibits Adiponectin Release from Human Adipose Tissue Explants and Adiposities. *Environ Health Perspect.* 2008 December; 116(12): 1642-1647http://www.ncbi.nlm.nih.gov/pmc/articles/PMC2599757/

Iqbal N et al: Effects of a Low-intensity Intervention That Prescribed a Low-carbohydrate vs. a Low-fat Diet in Obese, Diabetic Participants. *Obesity.* (2010) 18 9, 1733-1738. doi:10.1038/oby.2009.460 http://www.nature.com/oby/journal/v18/n9/full/oby2009460a.html

Jakicic JM et al: Effect of Exercise on 24-Month Weight Loss Maintenance in Overweight Women. John M. Arch Intern Med. 2008; 168(14):1550-1559. . http://archinte.ama-assn.org/cgi/content/abstract/168/14/1550

Johnston CS et al: Vinegar Improves Insulin Sensitivity to a High-Carbohydrate Meal in Subjects With Insulin Resistance or Type 2 Diabetes. *Diabetes Care.* 27:281-282, 2004 http://care.diabetesjournals.org/content/27/1/281.full

Johnston CS et al: Ketogenic low-carbohydrate diets have no metabolic advantage over nonketogenic low-carbohydrate diets. *Am J Clin Nutr.* May 2006 vol. 83 no. 5 1055-1061 http://www.ajcn.org/content/83/5/1055.full

Karakas SE et al: Relation of nutrients and hormones in polycystic ovary syndrome. *Am J Clin Nutr.* 2007; 685:688 -94. http://www.ajcn.org/content/85/3/688.abstract

Khan A: Insulin potentiating factor and chromium content of selected foods and spices. *Biol Trace Elem Res.* 1990 Mar; 24(3):183-8 http://www.ncbi.nlm.nih.gov/pubmed/1702671

Khaw K et al: Association of Hemoglobin A1C with Cardiovascular Disease and Mortality in Adults: The European Prospective Investigation into Cancer in Norfolk. *Annals of Internal Medicine.* 9/21/2004, Vol 141, no 6, 413-420 http://www.annals.org/content/141/6/413.abstract

Kim JH et al: Variations in conjugated linoleic acid (CLA) content of processed cheese by lactation time, feeding regimen, and ripening. *J Agric Food Chem.* 2009, 57 (8), pp 3235-3239 http://pubs.acs.org/doi/abs/10.1021/jf803838u

Kissileff HR et al: Leptin reverses declines in satiation in weight-reduced obese humans. *Am J Clin Nutr.* February 2012 vol. 95 no. 2 309-317 http://www.ajcn.org/content/95/2/309.abstract

Klöting N et al: Insulin-sensitive obesity. *AJP — Endo.* September 2010 vol. 299 no. 3 E506-E515 http://ajpendo.physiology.org/content/299/3/E506.full.pdf

Koh KK et al: Simvastatin Improves Flow-Mediated Dilation but Reduces Adiponectin Levels and Insulin Sensitivity in Hypercholesterolemic Patients. *Diabetes Care.* April 2008 vol. 31 no. 4 776-782 http://care.diabetesjournals.org/content/31/4/776.abstract

Kolata G: Putting Very Little Weight in Calorie Counting Methods. *New York Times.* 12/20/2007 http://www.nytimes.com/2007/12/20/health/nutrition/20BEST.html

Kopple JD: Do low-protein diets retard the loss of kidney function in patients with diabetic nephropathy? *Am J Clin Nutr.* Vol 88, No 3, 593-594, Sept 2008. http://www.ajcn.org/content/88/3/593.full

Kreider RB et al: Effects of Conjugated Linoleic Acid Supplementation During Resistance Training on Body Composition, Bone Density, Strength, and Selected Hematological Markers. *Journal of Strength & Conditioning Research.* August 2002 - Volume 16 - Issue 3 http://journals.lww.com/nsca-jscr/abstract/2002/08000/effects_of_conjugated_linoleic_acid.1.aspx

Kreitzman S et al: Glycogen storage: illusions of easy weight loss, excessive weight regain, and distortions in estimates of body composition. *Am J Clin Nutr.* July 1992 vol. 56 no. 1 292S-293S http://www.ajcn.org/content/56/1/292S.long

Kruszynska YT, et al,: In vivo regulation of liver and skeletal muscle glycogen synthase activity by glucose and insulin. *Diabetes.* June 1986 vol. 35 no. 6 662-667 http://diabetes.diabetesjournals.org/content/35/6/662.short

Larkin C: Lipitor Topped Worldwide Drug Sales in 2010; Crestor Gains Most. http://www.bloomberg.com/news/2011-02-10/lipitor-topped-worldwide-drug-sales-in-2010-crestor-gains-most.html

Laureys S: Residual Cerebral Functioning In The Vegetative State. Life-Sustaining Treatments And Vegetative State: Scientific advances and ethical dilemmas. 17-18-19-20 March, 2004 Rome, Italy http://www.timeoutintensiva.it/download/Laureys.pdf

Lazo M et al: Non-alcoholic fatty liver disease and mortality among US adults: prospective cohort study. Mariana *BMJ.* 2011; 343 http://www.bmj.com/content/343/bmj.d6891

Lê KA et al: Fructose over-consumption causes dyslipedemia and ectopic lipid deposition in healthy subjects with and without a family history of type 2 diabetes. L *Am J Clin Nutr.* 2009 Jun; 89(6):1760-5. Epub 2009 Apr 29 http://www.ncbi.nlm.nih.gov/pubmed/19403641

Lee J et al: Production of lipase-catalyzed structured lipids from safflower oil with conjugated linoleic acid and oxidation studies with rosemary extracts. *Food Research International*. Volume 37, Issue 10, 2004, Pages 967-974 http://www.sciencedirect.com/science/article/pii/S0963996904001450

Lim S et al: Chronic Exposure to the Herbicide, Atrazine, Causes Mitochondrial Dysfunction and Insulin Resistance. *PLoSOne*. Apr 13, 2009 http://www.plosone.org/article/info%3Adoi%2F10.1371%2Fjournal.pone.0005186

Lind MP et al: Circulating Levels of Phthalate Metabolites Are Associated With Prevalent Diabetes in the Elderly. *Diabetes Care*. Published online before print April 12, 2012 http://care.diabetesjournals.org/content/early/2012/04/11/dc11-2396

Loh K et al: Reactive Oxygen Species Enhance Insulin Sensitivity. *Cell Metabolism*.Volume 10, Issue 4, 260-272, 7 October 2009 http://www.ncbi.nlm.nih.gov/pmc/articles/PMC2892288/

Lopez-Ridaura R et al: Magnesium intake and risk of type 2 diabetes in men and women. *Diabetes Care*. 27:134-140, 2003 http://care.diabetesjournals.org/content/27/1/134.full

MacDonald M J. et al: Differences between human and rodent pancreatic islets: low pyruvate carboxylase, ATP citrate lyase and pyruvate carboxylation; high glucose-stimulated acetoacetate in human pancreatic islets. J *Biol Chem*. March 22, 2011 http://www.jbc.org/content/early/2011/03/22/jbc.M111.241182

MacDonald T: Recipes from the Wonderful Cooks at alt.support.diet.low-carb http://www.camacdonald.com/lc/LowCarbohydrateCooking-Recipes.htm

Mackay, EM et al: The Amount Of Water Stored With Glycogen In The Liver. *J Biol Chem*. 1934 105: 59-62 http://www.jbc.org/content/105/1/59.full.pdf

Manninen AH: Very-low-carbohydrate diets and preservation of muscle mass. *Nutr Metab*. 2006; 3: 9 http://www.ncbi.nlm.nih.gov/pmc/articles/PMC1373635/

Martin CK et al: Change in Food Cravings, Food Preferences, and Appetite During a Low-Carbohydrate and Low-Fat Diet. *Obesity*. 19, 1963-1970 (October 2011) http://www.nature.com/oby/journal/v19/n10/full/oby201162a.html

Martin SS et al: Apolipoprotein B but not LDL Cholesterol Is Associated With Coronary Artery Calcification in Type 2 Diabetic Whites. *Diabetes*. August 2009 vol. 58 no. 8 1887-1892 doi: 10.2337/db08-1794 http://diabetes.diabetesjournals.org/content/58/8/1887.abstract

Mavropoulos JC et al: The effects of a low-carbohydrate, ketogenic diet on the polycystic ovary syndrome: a pilot study. *Nutrition & Metabolism*. 2005, 2:35 http://www.biomedcentral.com/content/pdf/1743-7075-2-35.pdf

McAuley KA et al,: Long-term effects of popular dietary approaches on weight loss and features of insulin resistance. KA McAuley. *International Journal of Obesity*. (2006) 30, 342-349. http://www.nature.com/ijo/journal/v30/n2/pdf/0803075a.pdf

McAuley KA et al: Comparison of high-fat and high-protein diets with a high-carbohydrate diet in insulin-resistant obese women. K. A. *Diabetologia*. (2005) 48: 8-16 http://www.springerlink.com/content/1abv5hablr8veyrm/fulltext.pdf

McDonald, L, *The Ketogenic Diet*. Austin TX, ISBN 0-9671456-0-0, 1998. http://books.google.com/books?id=JtCZBe-2XVIC

Mead NM: Programmed Obesity?: Study Links Intrauterine Exposures to Higher BMI in Toddlers. *Environ Health Perspect*. 2009 January; 117(1): A33. http://www.ncbi.nlm.nih.gov/pmc/articles/PMC2627889/

Medscape Family Medicine: FDA Warns Doctors, Consumers About Red Yeast Supplements Found to Contain Lovastatin. http://www.medscape.com/viewarticle/561289?sssdmh=dm1.293361

Mekary RA et al: Physical Activity in Relation to Long-term Weight Maintenance After Intentional Weight Loss in Premenopausal Women. *Obesity*. (2010) 18 1, 167-174 http://www.nature.com/oby/journal/v18/n1/abs/oby2009170a.html

The Merck Manuel: Hypoglycemia http://www.merckmanuals.com/home/hormonal_and_metabolic_disorders/hypoglycemia/hypoglycemia.html

Mesci B et al: Dietary Breads Myth or Reality. *Diabetes Research and Clinical Practice*. Volume 81, Issue 1, July 2008, Pages 68-71 http://www.sciencedirect.com/science/article/pii/S0168822708000934

Nachman F et al: Gastroesophageal Reflux Symptoms in Patients With Celiac Disease and the Effects of a Gluten-Free Diet. *Clinical Gastroenterology and Hepatology*. Volume 9, Issue 3 , Pages 214-219, March 2011 http://www.cghjournal.org/article/S1542-3565(10)00661-0/abstract

Neighmond P: Weight-Loss Surgery: It's Not for Everyone. Aug 17, 2006 http://www.npr.org/templates/story/story.php?storyId=5658690

Nielsen JV et al: A low-carbohydrate diet may prevent end-stage renal failure in type 2 diabetes. A case report. *Nutr Metab* . 2006; 3: 23 http://www.ncbi.nlm.nih.gov/pmc/articles/PMC1523335/

NIH: National Diabetes Statistics, 2011. http://diabetes.niddk.nih.gov/dm/pubs/statistics/#NewCasesDDY20

Nilsson L et al: Liver and Muscle Glycogen in Man after Glucose and Fructose Infusion. *Scandinavian Journal of Clinical & Laboratory Investigation*. 1974, Vol. 33, No. 1, Pages 5-10 http://informahealthcare.com/doi/abs/10.3109/00365517409114190

Nilsson LH: Liver Glycogen in Man-the Effect of Total Starvation or a Carbohydrate-Poor Diet Followed by Carbohydrate Refeeding. *Scandinavian Journal of Clinical & Laboratory Investigation*. 1973, Vol. 32, No. 4 , Pages 325-330 http://informahealthcare.com/doi/abs/10.3109/00365517309084355

Nuttall FQ et al: Glycemic Response to Ingested Dreamfields Pasta Compared With Traditional Pasta. *Diabetes Care*. January 26, 2011 vol. 34 no. 2 e17-e18 Withdrawn. http://care.diabetesjournals.org/content/34/2/e17.full

Olsen DE et al: Screening for Diabetes and Pre-Diabetes With Proposed A1C-Based Diagnostic Criteria. *Diabetes Care*. October 2010 vol. 33 no. 10 2184-2189 http://care.diabetesjournals.org/content/33/10/2184.abstract

Owen OE: Brain Metabolism during Fasting. *J Clin Inv*. Vol. 46, Nov. 10, 1967 http://www.ncbi.nlm.nih.gov/pmc/articles/PMC292907/pdf/jcinvest00272-0077.pdf

Paleohacks: Is lowered T3 resulting from a low carb diet problematic? http://paleohacks.com/questions/78343/is-lowered-t3-resulting-from-a-low-carb-diet-problematic

Pan Y et al: Low-protein diet for diabetic nephropathy: a meta-analysis of randomized controlled trials. *Am J Clin Nutr*. Vol. 88, No. 3, 660-666, September 2008 http://www.ajcn.org/content/88/3/660.abstract

Pasquali R et al: Effect of dietary carbohydrates during hypocaloric treatment of obesity on peripheral thyroid hormone metabolism. *J Endocrinol Invest*. 1982 Jan-Feb; 5(1):47-52 http://www.ncbi.nlm.nih.gov/pubmed/7096916

Patel AM et al: Got Calcium? Welcome to the Calcium-Alkali Syndrome Ami M. Patel and Stanley Goldfarb. *J Am Soc Nephrol*. 21: 1440-1443, 2010 http://jasn.asnjournals.org/content/21/9/1440.abstract

Patten SB et al: Major Depression, Antidepressant Medication and the Risk of Obesity. *Psychother Psychosom*. 2009; 78:182-186 http://content.karger.com/ProdukteDB/produkte.asp?doi=10.1159/000209349

Perley, MJ et al: Plasma Insulin Responses to Oral and Intravenous Glucose: Studies in Normal and Diabetic Subjects. *J Clin Invest*. 1967 December; 46(12): 1954-1962. http://www.ncbi.nlm.nih.gov/pmc/articles/PMC292948/pdf/jcinvest00274-0088.pdf

Persaud SJ et al: Gymnema sylvestre stimulates insulin release in vitro by increased membrane permeability. *J Endocrinol*. November 1, 1999 163 207-212 http://joe.endocrinology-journals.org/content/163/2/207.full.pdf

Petersen KF et al:Impaired mitochondrial activity in the insulin-resistant offspring of patients with type 2 diabetes. *New England J Med*. 2004 Feb 12; 350(7); 639-41 http://www.nejm.org/doi/full/10.1056/NEJMoa031314

Piconi S et al: Treatment of periodontal disease results in improvements in endothelial dysfunction and reduction of the carotid intima-media thickness. *FASEB Journal*. December 12, 2008, vol. 23 no. 4 1196-1204 http://www.fasebj.org/content/23/4/1196.abstract

Poplawski MM et al: Reversal of Diabetic Nephropathy by a Ketogenic Diet. *PLoS ONE*. 2011; 6 http://www.plosone.org/article/info%3Adoi%2F10.1371%2Fjournal.pone.0018604

Rabast U, et al: Loss of weight, sodium and water in obese persons consuming a high- or low-carbohydrate diet. *Ann Nutr Metab*. 1981; 25(6):341-9.http://www.ncbi.nlm.nih.gov/pubmed/7332312

Raff M et al: Conjugated Linoleic Acids Reduce Body Fat in Healthy Postmenopausal Women, *J Nutr*. July 2009 vol. 139 no. 7 1347-1352 http://jn.nutrition.org/content/139/7/1347.full.pdf

Ramkuma KM et al: Inhibitory effect of Gymnema Montanum leaves on a-glucosidase activity and a-amylase activity and their relationship with polyphenolic content. *Medicinal Chemistry Research*. Volume 19, Number 8, (2010) 948-961 http://www.springerlink.com/content/3v64u63872m24l38/

Ren X et al: Sweet taste signaling functions as a hypothalamic glucose sensor. *Front Integr Neurosci*. 3:12. 2009 http://frontiersin.org/integrativeneuroscience/paper/10.3389/neuro.07/012.2009/html/

Risérus U et al: Supplementation With Conjugated Linoleic Acid Causes Isomer-Dependent Oxidative Stress and Elevated C-Reactive Protein: A Potential Link to Fatty Acid-Induced Insulin Resistance. *Circulation*. 2002; 106: 1925-1929. http://www.ncbi.nlm.nih.gov/pubmed/12370214

Risérus U, et al: Conjugated linoleic acid (CLA) reduced abdominal adipose tissue in obese middle-aged men with signs of the metabolic syndrome: a randomised controlled trial. International Journal of Obesity and Related Metabolic Disorders. *Journal of the International Association for the Study of Obesity*. 2001, 25(8):1129-35 http://ukpmc.ac.uk/abstract/MED/11477497

Rosenbaum M et al: Long-term persistence of adaptive thermogenesis in subjects who have maintained a reduced body weight. *Am J Clin Nutr*. October 2008 vol. 88 no. 4 906-912 http://www.ajcn.org/content/88/4/906.long

Rotshteyn Y et al: Application of modified in vitro screening procedure for identifying herbals possessing sulfonylurea-like activity. *Journal of Ethnopharmacology.* Volume 93, Issues 2-3, August 2004, Pages 337-344 http://www.sciencedirect.com/science/article/pii/S0378874104001795

Rubin RR et al: Elevated Depression Symptoms, Antidepressant Medicine Use, and Risk of Developing Diabetes During the Diabetes Prevention Program. *Diabetes Care.* 31:420-426, 2008 http://care.diabetesjournals.org/content/31/3/420.abstract

Ruhl, Jenny. *Blood Sugar 101: What They Don't Tell You About Diabetes.* Technion Books, Turners Falls, MA. ISBN 978-0-9647116-1-7

Sachdeva A et al: Lipid levels in patients hospitalized with coronary artery disease: An analysis of 136,905 hospitalizations in Get With The Guidelines. *American Heart Journal.* Volume 157, Issue 1 , Pages 111-117.e2, January 2009 http://www.ahjonline.com/article/S0002-8703(08)00717-5/abstract

Sanders KM et al: Annual High-Dose Oral Vitamin D and Falls and Fractures in Older Women. *JAMA.* 2010; 303(18):1815-1822. http://jama.ama-assn.org/content/303/18/1815.abstract

Science Daily: Leptin Has Powerful Effect On Reward Center In The Brain. http://www.sciencedaily.com/releases/2006/09/060929094058.htm

Science Daily: Toxic Plastics: Bisphenol A Linked To Metabolic Syndrome In Human Tissue http://www.sciencedaily.com/releases/2008/09/080904151629.htm

Sclafani A: Sweet taste signaling in the gut. *PNAS.* September 18, 2007 vol. 104 no. 38 14887-14888 http://www.pnas.org/content/104/38/14887.full

Selvin E et al: Glycated Hemoglobin, Diabetes and Cardiovascular Risk in Nondiabetic Adults. *NEJM.* Volume 362:800-811. March 4, 2010 Number 9.http://www.nejm.org/doi/full/10.1056/NEJMoa0908359

Selvin E et al: Glycemic Control and Coronary Heart Disease Risk in Persons With and Without Diabetes. The Atherosclerosis Risk in Communities Study. *Arch Intern Med.* 2005; 165:1910-1916. http://www.ncbi.nlm.nih.gov/pubmed/16157837?dopt=Abstract

Sesso HD et al: Vitamins E and C in the Prevention of Cardiovascular Disease in Men. The Physicians' Health Study II Randomized Controlled Trial. *JAMA.* 2008; 300(18):2123-2133 http://jama.ama-assn.org/content/300/18/2123.long

Shaham O et al: Metabolic profiling of the human response to a glucose challenge reveals distinct axes of insulin sensitivity. *Mol Syst Biol.* 2008; 4:214. Epub 2008 Aug 5. ttp://www.ncbi.nlm.nih.gov/pubmed/18682704

Shai I et al: Weight Loss with a Low-Carbohydrate, Mediterranean, or Low-Fat Diet. *N Engl J Med.* 2008; 359:229-241 http://www.nejm.org/doi/full/10.1056/NEJMoa0708681

Shomon M: Top Doctors http://www.thyroid-info.com/topdrs/index.htm

Singh RB et al: Effect of hydrosoluble coenzyme Q10 on blood pressures and insulin resistance in hypertensive patients with coronary artery disease. *Journal of Human Hypertension.* (1999) 13, 203-208 www.ncbi.nlm.nih.gov/pubmed/10204818

Sisson M: *The Primal Blueprint: Reprogram your genes for effortless weight loss, vibrant health, and boundless energy.* Primal Nutrition, Inc.; 2nd ed, 2012. ISBN-13: 978-0982207789

Snopes: Death of a Diet Doctor. http://www.snopes.com/medical/doctor/atkins.asp

Song Y et al: Dietary magnesium intake in relation to plasma insulin levels and risk of type 2 diabetes in women. *Diabetes Care.* 27:59-65, 2003 http://www.ncbi.nlm.nih.gov/pubmed/14693967

Spijkerman AM et al: Microvascular complications at time of diagnosis of type 2 diabetes are similar among diabetic patients detected by targeted screening and patients newly diagnosed in general practice: the hoorn screening study. *Diabetes Care.* 2003 Sep; 26(9):2604-8. http://www.ncbi.nlm.nih.gov/pubmed/12941726

Stevens A et al: Sudden Cardiac Death of an Adolescent During Dieting. *Southern Medical Journal.* September 2002 - Volume 95 - Issue 9 http://journals.lww.com/smajournalonline/Abstract/2002/09000/Sudden_Cardiac_Death_of_an_Adolescent_During.23.aspx

Stock S, et al: Ghrelin, peptide YY, glucose-dependent insulinotropic polypeptide, and hunger responses to a mixed meal in anorexic, obese, and control female adolescents. *J Clin Endocrinol Metab.* 2005 Apr; 90(4):2161-8. Epub 2005 Jan 18. http://www.ncbi.nlm.nih.gov/pubmed/15657373

St-Onge M-P et al: Greater rise in fat oxidation with medium-chain triglyceride consumption relative to long-chain triglyceride is associated with lower initial body weight and greater loss of subcutaneous adipose tissue. *International Journal of Obesity.* (Sept 2003) 27, 1565-1571. http://www.nature.com/ijo/journal/v27/n12/abs/0802467a.html

St-Onge M-P et al: Medium Chain Triglyceride Oil Consumption as Part of a Weight Loss Diet Does Not Lead to an Adverse Metabolic Profile When Compared to Olive Oil. *J Am Coll Nutr.* October 2008 vol. 27 no. 5 547-552 http://www.jacn.org/content/27/5/547.short

St-Onge M-P et al: Medium-Chain Triglycerides Increase Energy Expenditure and Decrease Adiposity in Overweight Men. *Obesity Research*. Vol. 11 No. 3 March 2003 http://www.absoluteorganix.co.za/mct1.pdf

Straczkowski M et al: Insulin resistance in the first-degree relatives of persons with Type 2 Diabetes. *Med Sci Monit*. 2003 May; 9(5):CR186-90. http://www.ncbi.nlm.nih.gov/pubmed/12761455?dopt=Abstract

Stranges S et al: Effects of Long-Term Selenium Supplementation on the Incidence of Type 2 Diabetes: A Randomized Trial. *Annals of Internal Medicine*. Volume 147, no. 4 (2007) 217-223 http://www.annals.org/content/147/4/217.full

Suzuki S et al: The effects of coenzyme Q10 treatment on maternally inherited diabetes mellitus and deafness, and mitochondrial DNA 3243 (A to G) mutation. S. Suzuki, *Diabetologia*. (1998) 41: 584-588 http://www.ncbi.nlm.nih.gov/pubmed/9628277

Tai K et al: Glucose tolerance and vitamin D: Effects of treating vitamin D deficiency. *Nutrition*. Volume 24, Issue 10, Pages 950-956 (October 2008) http://www.nutritionjrnl.com/article/S0899-9007(08)00205-0/abstract

Teeuw WJ et al: Effect of Periodontal Treatment on Glycemic Control of Diabetic Patients: A systematic review and meta-analysis. *Diabetes Care*. February 2010 vol. 33 no. 2 421-427 doi: 10.2337/dc09-1378 http://care.diabetesjournals.org/content/33/2/421.abstract

Teitlebaum SL et al: Associations between phthalate metabolite urinary concentrations and body size measures in New York City children. Environmental Research.Volume 112, January 2012, Pages 186–193 http://www.sciencedirect.com/science/article/pii/S0013935111003112

Tendler D et al: The Effect of a Low-Carbohydrate, Ketogenic Diet on Nonalcoholic Fatty Liver Disease: A Pilot Study. *Digestive Diseases and Sciences*. Vol. 52, No. 2, (2007) 589-593, http://www.springerlink.com/content/r5170lh8532t7452/

Tirosh A:Normal fasting plasma glucose levels and type 2 diabetes in young men. *N Engl J Med*. 2005 Oct 6;353(14):1454-62 http://www.ncbi.nlm.nih.gov/pubmed/16207847

The Whole Grains Council: http://www.wholegrainscouncil.org/whole-grains-101/health-studies-on-whole-grains

Thompson D J et al: Effect of Monosodium Glutamate on Blood Ketones in Sheep. *J Nutrition*. 1968, 96: 415-420. http://jn.nutrition.org/content/96/3/415.full.pdf

Törnkvist A et al: PCDD/F, PCB, PBDE, HBCD and chlorinated pesticides in a Swedish market basket from 2005 - Levels and dietary intake estimations. *Chemosphere*. Volume 83, Issue 2, March 2011, Pages 193-199 http://www.sciencedirect.com/science/article/pii/S0045653510014475

Tremblay E: Thermogenesis and weight loss in obese individuals: a primary association with organochlorine pollution. *International Journal of Obesity* (2004) 28, 936–939 http://www.nature.com/ijo/journal/v28/n7/full/0802527a.html

USDA Food Safety and Inspection Service: Home / Science / Data Collection & Reports / Chemistry http://www.fsis.usda.gov/science/chemistry/index.asp

Van der Vies J: Two Methods for the Determination of Glycogen in Liver. *Biochem J*. 1954 July; 57(3): 410-416. http://www.ncbi.nlm.nih.gov/pmc/articles/PMC1269772/pdf/biochemj01083-0061.pdf

Vanschoonbeek K et al: Cinnamon supplementation does not improve glycemic control in postmenopausal type 2 diabetes patients. *J Nutr*. 2006 Apr; 136(4):977-80 http://www.ncbi.nlm.nih.gov/pubmed/16549460?dopt=abstract

Villani RG et al: L-Carnitine supplementation combined with aerobic training does not promote weight loss in moderately obese women. *Int J Sport Nutr Exerc Metab*. 2000 Jun; 10(2):199-207 http://www.ncbi.nlm.nih.gov/pubmed/10861338

Vinson JA et al: Investigation of an Amylase Inhibitor on Human Glucose Absorption after Starch Consumption. *The Open Nutraceuticals Journal*. 2009, 2, 88-91 http://www.benthamscience.com/open/tonutraj/articles/V002/88TONUTRAJ.pdf

Volek JS et al: Cardiovascular and Hormonal Aspects of Very-Low-Carbohydrate Ketogenic Diets. *Obesity*. (2004) 12, 115S-123S http://www.nature.com/oby/journal/v12/n11s/full/oby2004276a.html

Volek JS et al: Comparison of a Very Low-Carbohydrate and Low-Fat Diet on Fasting Lipids, LDL Subclasses, Insulin Resistance, and Postprandial Lipemic Responses in Overweight Women. *J Am Coll Nutr*. April 2004 vol. 23 no. 2 177-184 http://www.jacn.org/content/23/2/177.full

Volek JS et al: *The New Atkins for a New You: The Ultimate Diet for Shedding Weight and Feeling Great*. Touchstone, New York, 2010, ISBN: 978143919027.

Wadden TA et al: Four-Year Weight Losses in the Look AHEAD Study: Factors Associated with Long-Term Success. *Obesity*. (Silver Spring). 2011 October; 19(10): 1987-1998 http://www.ncbi.nlm.nih.gov/pmc/articles/PMC3183129/

Westman EC et al:The effect of a low-carbohydrate, ketogenic diet versus a low-glycemic index diet on gly-cemic control in type 2 diabetes mellitus. *Nutrition & Metabolism*. 2008, 5:36 doi:10.1186/1743-7075-5-36 http://www.nutritionandmetabolism.com/content/5/1/36

White AM et al: Vinegar Ingestion at Bedtime Moderates Waking Glucose Concentrations in Adults With Well-Controlled Type 2 Diabetes. *Diabetes Care*. November 2007 vol. 30 no. 11 2814-2815. http://care.diabetesjournals.org/content/30/11/2814.full

Whole Health Source: Can Vitamin K2 Reverse Arterial Calcification? http://wholehealthsource.blogspot.com/2008/11/can-vitamin-k2-reverse-arterial.html

Wikipedia: Brain http://en.wikipedia.org/wiki/Human_brain#Metabolism

Wikipedia: Glycogen http://en.wikipedia.org/wiki/Glycogen

Wing RR et al: A Self-Regulation Program for Maintenance of Weight Loss. Rena R. Wing. *N Engl J Med*. 2006; 355:1563-1571 October 12, 2006 http://www.nejm.org/doi/full/10.1056/NEJMoa061883

Wing RR et al: Long-term weight loss maintenance. *American Journal of Clinical Nutrition*. Vol. 82, No. 1, 222S-225S, July 2005 http://www.ajcn.org/content/82/1/222S.long

Witham MD, et al: The effect of different doses of vitamin D(3) on markers of vascular health in patients with type 2 diabetes: a randomised controlled trial. *Diabetologia*. 2010 Oct; 53(10):2112-9. http://www.ncbi.nlm.nih.gov/pubmed/20596692

Wolever TMS: Sugar Alcohols and Diabetes: A Review. *Canadian Journal of Diabetes*. 2002; 26(4):356-362. P. 5 http://www.diabetes.ca/Files/SugarAlcohols-Wolever-CJDDecember2002.pdf

Yancy WS et al: A Low-Carbohydrate, Ketogenic Diet versus a Low-Fat Diet To Treat Obesity and Hyperlipi-demia. A Randomized, Controlled Trial. *Ann Int Med*. May 18, 2004 vol. 140 no. 10 769-77 http://www.annals.org/content/140/10/769.full

Yang H: Increased Mortality Risk for Cancers of the Kidney and Other Urinary Organs among Chinese Herbal-ists. *Journal of Epidemiology*. Vol. 19 (2009) , No. 1 pp.17-23 http://www.jstage.jst.go.jp/article/jea/19/1/19_17/_article

Yin X: Ghrelin fluctuation, what determines its production? Xuefeng Yin Acta Biochim *Biophys Sin*. (2009) 41 (3): 188-197. http://abbs.oxfordjournals.org/content/41/3/188.full.pdf

Zipitis CS, et al: Vitamin D supplementation in early childhood and risk of type 1 diabetes: a systematic review and meta-analysis. *Archives of Disease in Childhood*. 2008; 93:512-517 http://care.diabetesjournals.org/content/33/9/1962.abstract

Index

Z